Other titles in *The Daily Telegraph* series

To order further health titles from Robinson,
please see the order form at the back of this book.

The Daily Telegraph

HOME DOCTOR

The Complete Guide to Treating
Common Conditions at Home

Dr Caroline Shreeve

ROBINSON
London

Constable & Robinson Ltd
3 The Lanchesters
162 Fulham Palace Road
London W6 9ER
www.constablerobinson.com

First published in the UK by Robinson,
an imprint of Constable & Robinson Ltd 2005

Publishers Note: This book is intended as a general reference book
and a manual for self-treatment. The information given here is
designed to help you make informed choices about your health. It is
by no means intended as a substitute for any treatment prescribed by
your doctor.

ISBN 1-84529-099-2

Printed and bound in the EU.

1 3 5 7 9 10 8 6 4 2

This book is dedicated with lots of love to Marilyn Evans, stalwart ally in adversity and the source of the most wonderful, shared laughter.

Contents

Foreword
by Dr James Le Fanu

The workings of the human body are proving to be more wonderful and mysterious than anyone could have imagined. As Caroline Shreeve points out, electrical monitoring has identified no less than 4,000 previously unrecognized 'potent points' on the surface of the skin. These are highly sensitive to bioelectrical charges and thus provide a plausible rationale for the many therapeutic benefits of the traditional Chinese therapy of acupuncture. Similarly physiological investigation of those practising the traditional Indian movement therapy, yoga, has confirmed their ability to influence those 'automatic' bodily functions such as heartbeat, temperature control and blood pressure, previously thought to be not amenable to conscious control.

The profound implications of such findings scarcely need spelling out. They challenge western science's assumption of an exclusive claim to understanding the mechanisms of human biology. It is now possible to see how the undoubtedly spectacular success of western medicine over the last forty years has nonetheless been at the cost of a narrowing of vision and as a result a failure to recognize the many homoeostatic and healing mechanisms that form the basis of the complementary therapies.

Caroline Shreeve's special insight, which makes her book so invaluable, is that many of these therapies, not just acupuncture and yoga, but herbal medicine, aromatherapy and homoeopathy are particularly suitable for self-treatment thus markedly extending the range of therapeutic options for a whole range of ailments.

The options for treatment in sinusitis, for example, extend well beyond the standard medical treatment of steam inhalation and antibiotics, to include dietary advice to reduce the intake of meat and dairy foods thus (for reasons unknown) inhibiting mucus production; decongestant essential oils such as eucalyptus and tea tree oil; ginger root and ginseng to combat infection; acupuncture *and* two specific yoga positions, Corpse and Shoulder Stand.

These multi-treatment options for sinusitis illustrate an important point that perhaps should be better understood. The complementary therapies are, in a sense, complementary to each other as well as mainstream medicine, working in different ways to achieve the same end. While each alone may not work in every case, still it would be expected that combined they would have a cumulative effect.

The progressive incorporation of the complementary therapies into mainstream medicine is one of the most striking developments in recent years. It would not be unreasonable to imagine that in a decade or so, most family doctors at least will have a book just like this on their desk to consult when advising their patients on the best treatment for their ailments. Those who buy this book will not have to wait that long – with the added bonus they do not even have to bother their doctor – but can get on with treating themselves in the more salubrious surroundings of their own home.

Introduction

'Why bother the doctor?' is a familiar response of people who privately recognize their need for treatment but dislike asking for it. The refrain now has a healthier ring – the doctor's surgery often *can* be safely avoided if you can identify common complaints, know what to do about them and maybe prevent them altogether.

Both orthodox and complementary medicines are accessible from a wide range of sources – from the internet, supermarkets and corner shops to pharmacies, qualified therapists and health-food stores. The purpose of this book is to enable to you recognize everyday disorders that we all encounter in ourselves, families and friends, and to select one or more treatments to suit personal needs.

Complementary treatments are becoming steadily more popular and, if used wisely, are both effective and safe. Most marry happily with orthodox medicine and many doctors nowadays encourage their use. In fact growing numbers of GPs themselves study and practise the therapies and willingly co-operate with holistic practitioners when asked to do so.

Herbal medicine, aromatherapy, homoeopathic medicine, acupuncture, Yoga and relaxation are no longer 'fringe' subjects. Self-treatment – either with them or with conventional over-the-counter medicines – is rapidly becoming a matter of necessity because of the interminable wait many of us experience for out-patient and health-centre appointments. Even if this were not the case, it is far more convenient, comfortable and satisfying to deal with minor ailments at home, where access to remedies can be re-assuringly immediate.

Nutritional medicine is mentioned in every case, since vitality and well-being cannot possibly peak without an ongoing supply of essential nutrients. Cutting down our intake of saturated fat and salt, for example, reduces our risks of heart disease, obesity and stroke. It also lessens the financial toll upon the National Health Service. But, worthy as this aim surely is, a much more attractive reason exists for eating healthily. Avoiding known dietary hazards and choosing foods that supply our nutritional needs helps us steer clear of many grave disorders. It also increases energy and stamina, boosts the immune defence system against cancer, infectious illnesses, premature ageing and allergies, and enhances the condition of both body and mind.

Herbal medicines are also mentioned in most instances, as are aromatherapy oils, homoeopathic remedies, relaxation exercises and acupressure techniques. Each has its part to play in relieving particular ailments and some will appeal to you more than others. None, however, should be used indiscriminately or in any way other than as directed on the packaging.

Standardized herbal medicines manufactured by reputable companies are safe and reliable, but clearly if they are potent enough to help you to sleep or quell an attack of diarrhoea, for instance, they are equally capable of harming you if you ignore the label instructions. The same principle applies, of course, to the drug remedies listed for every entry. Even gentle acupressure can have highly potent effects and the use of a number of techniques is advised against during pregnancy.

I must also mention that this book is no substitute for consulting a qualified practitioner – family doctor or complementary therapist – when the need exists.

How to Use this Book

Part I provides an overview of the key complementary therapies that can help you maintain good health and treat specific illnesses. Part II provides a detailed step-by-step guide to treatment.

Details of every ailment included here are given to help you decide what you are dealing with and how it should be treated. At the same time, each entry includes a section explaining how and when a visit to your local surgery becomes necessary.

Complementary Therapies and Treatments

1

Nutritional Medicine

MOST OF US know the ground rules for healthy eating. Fresh natural foods are fundamental to immune resistance and, by that token, to vitality and well-being. Fresh fruit and vegetables and their juices, lean meat and fish, soya, eggs and low-fat dairy products, grains, pulses, nuts and seeds all supply nutrients or plant medicines to meet particular needs. Freshly squeezed cabbage juice relieves mouth ulcers and an inflamed stomach, for instance, while oats reduce LDL (low-density lipoprotein) cholesterol and promote a healthy circulation, and turkey, cottage cheese, duck and avocado pears supply tryptophan, an amino acid that depression sufferers particularly need.

Antioxidants are particularly important. These are vitamins, minerals and trace elements that strengthen the immune system against free radicals – supercharged oxygen molecules which damage tissue when present in high numbers. Stress, 'trans' fatty acids (SEE *Fats and Oils*), viral illnesses, growing older, environmental radiation and atmospheric pollutants all encourage free radical production, which has been linked with allergies and impaired immunity, premature ageing and degenerative disorders such as cardiovascular disease, arthritis and cancer.

To combat this, five or more 100 g (4 oz) daily portions of fresh fruit and vegetables are traditionally recommended. Health experts disagree over whether nutritional supplements are also required. Studies have indicated that such supplements can increase cancer risks, however a number of nutritionists still approve of them, albeit in smaller quantities, and it's worth bearing in mind that the nutritional value of many greengrocery products has dropped since the 1950s. A satisfactory compromise seems to be a mainly wholefood diet with a wide choice of plant foods, periodically supplemented with additional nutrients.

Even small concessions to improved nutrition bring significant benefits. Replacing at least some refined white flour and sugar with whole cereals, grains and fresh and dried fruit helps to normalize blood sugar levels and prevent arterial disease and cancer. Reducing total fat and replacing butter and lard with plant oils rich in polyunsaturates will reduce blood cholesterol and the risks of developing arterial disease and cancer. Lean meat and poultry, fish, eggs, soya, pulses and nuts provide healthy protein low in saturated fat; eating less salt helps to reduce high blood pressure.

Carbohydrates, Fruit and Vegetables

Carbohydrates and foods providing them in significant quantities are classified according to their effects on the blood sugar level, on a scale known as the glycaemic index (GI). High GI items include unhealthy sugar-rich snacks and fast foods as well as healthier wholefoods (SEE *list on page 6*). Generally low in fibre, they send the blood sugar soaring, which in turn triggers the release of large quantities of insulin from the pancreas to drive the blood sugar into the cells. Two problems can arise from this – hypoglycaemia (low blood sugar), in response to the large volumes of released insulin, and insulin resistance. The former causes shakiness, a fast pulse, fears of collapse and sweating, and can be remedied by taking a little sugar and avoiding hot stuffy atmospheres. Insulin resistance increases the risks of diabetes and decreases the rate at which the body utilizes food fuel for energy, changing it instead into fat. Raised insulin levels are therefore linked with obesity and cardiovascular disease, heart attacks and strokes.

Low GI foods do the opposite: rich in fibre, they help to normalize blood glucose and insulin levels, thereby reducing the risks of diabetes and obesity, and prompting the body to burn fat. In addition, by lowering total and LDL (harmful) cholesterol, and raising the high-density lipoprotein (HDL, the type of cholesterol that helps to prevent arterial clogging and cuts the risk of heart attacks and strokes); low GIs cut the risk of heart attacks and strokes.

Low GI carbohydrates/fruit and vegetables

Breads: Multigrain white and brown breads, heavy fruit breads, oatcakes

Grains and breakfast cereals: Brown rice, wild rice, other wholegrains, pearl barley, tabbouleh, wholewheat pasta, unsweetened muesli, oats/porridge, high fibre wheatbran cereal

Vegetables: Okra, sweet potatoes, mushrooms, legumes (peas, beans), aubergines, artichokes, broccoli

Fruit: Apples, pears, mandarins, oranges, grapefruit, bananas

Other: Some low sugar/high fruit jams, unrefined honey, soya milk and its products

Intermediate GI carbohydrates

Breads: Light rye bread, pitta bread, sourdough bread

Grains and breakfast cereals: Long grain rice, white pasta, wholegrain wheat cereal bisks

Vegetables: Potatoes

Fruit: Strawberries, plums, raisins, red/black/whitecurrants

High GI carbohydrates

Breads: Wholegrain bread, white bread

Grains and breakfast cereals: Short grain rice, toasted rice cereal

Vegetables: Instant potato, tomatoes, lettuce, peppers, red cabbage, marrow

Fruit: Dried dates, watermelon

Other: Soft drinks, most confectionery

Especially beneficial...

Blueberries

Blueberries and their European counterparts, bilberries, have been used worldwide for centuries to treat poor eyesight, liver and lung disorders, digestive tract inflammation, mouth ulcers, piles, swollen legs and feet, and general bruising. Their chief active constituent is a group of antioxidants called anthocyanosides, which are concentrated in the skin of the fruit and responsible for its bluish-purple colour. At least fifteen different types of anthocyanosides have been identified, and their effectiveness is partly due to their enhancement of the 'microcirculation', i.e. capillary blood flow, notably in the eyes, the lungs and digestive tract and connective tissue.

Anthocyanosides also cut the risk of heart attacks and strokes, and combat cancer and age-related brain changes such as dementia, Alzheimer's disease and poor memory, concentration and co-ordination.

Blueberries also have an anti-bacterial action within the urinary tract, preventing organisms from sticking to the lining membranes and thereby relieving or helping to prevent cystitis and kidney infections.

The recommended daily intake of blueberries – around one handful (50–75 g or 2–3 oz) – can be mixed with breadcrumbs and herbs to flavour stuffing, blended with dairy or soya milk into a shake or smoothie, or added to yoghurt, muesli, porridge or other cereal, milk puddings, fruit compotes or savoury grain dishes such as rice or cous cous.

Broccoli

Broccoli was grown for medicinal purposes in medieval times and it is now proven to boost the immune system against cancer. Sulforaphane, a major player among broccoli's powerful constituents, mobilizes cellular enzymes that inactivate carcinogens and other foreign substances. And in the year 2000, scientists at the John Innes Centre in Norwich created a new non-GM 'super-broccoli' with up to 100 times more sulforaphane by crossing the normal plant with its wild Sicilian cousin.

Broccoli contains isothiocyanates, which trigger the manufacture of the body's own cancer-fighting chemicals and inhibit cellular growth in the skin cancer melanoma. A further constituent, indole-3-carbinol, cuts the risks of hormone-linked cancers of the breast, ovaries and prostate.

Broccoli and other cruciferous vegetables (those bearing cross-shaped flowers), for example Brussels sprouts, cabbage, kale, turnips and cauliflower, provide vitamin C; calcium, magnesium and other nutrients for strong teeth and bones, manganese for a prompt memory and strong muscles, and vitamin K, for normal blood clotting. They also reduce the risks of cataracts and certain birth defects and keep the heart and blood vessels healthy.

Oats

Oats contain the soluble fibre beta-glucan which, according to four decades of research, can combat blood clot (thrombus) formation and lower raised blood cholesterol by up to 23 per cent (a fall of 1 per cent is equivalent to a 2 per cent fall in the risk of heart disease). A medium-sized bowl of porridge daily is generally sufficient to achieve this. Alternatively, you could mix the same quantity of porridge oats with fresh or dried fruit, juice, nuts, seeds, wheatgerm or yoghurt to make muesli, or snack on oatcakes.

Oats also provide iron for a healthy brain and red blood cells, magnesium for normal heart function, zinc for wound healing, good eyesight and to combat colds and flu, the B vitamins thiamine and niacin, and antioxidants, vitamin E and bioflavonoids (SEE *below*).

Oats are also used in herbal medicine for their antidepressant effect and as a nerve tonic.

Oranges

Oranges have nearly 200 active plant chemicals, most significantly vitamin C and the bioflavonoids. These two potent antioxidants work synergistically (achieving more in combination than each working separately) to protect various tissues and organs from cancer, inflammation, infection, blood clots and the fatty deposits that clog arteries. They combat or reduce the risks of cancer, colds, flu and other infections, arthritis, asthma, heart attacks and strokes, high blood pressure and arterial disease. Other disorders thought to benefit from eating oranges include dementia, macular degeneration, gallstones, diabetes, cataracts and gum inflammation (gingivitis).

Hesperetin, a bioflavonoid in oranges, grapefruit and lemons, reduces high blood pressure, raises healthy HDL cholesterol and reduces the unhealthy LDL type. Herperidin, another bioflavonoid found in the peel, pith and white membranes of oranges, adds anti-inflammatory action to these benefits. Limonene, another citrus peel constituent, reduces the risks of squamous cell carcinoma of the skin, lungs and other organs. Ensure your intake of these nutrients with a fresh orange and/or grapefruit daily, and include some peel and pith when juicing.

Pumpkins

Pumpkins are very low in fat and calories and rich in soluble fibre. Their deep orange colour (like that of carrots, orange peppers and sweet potatoes) is due to high concentrations of alpha- and beta-carotene pigments (both forms of pro-vitamin A). Working with other antioxidants such as iron, potassium, folic acid, zinc, calcium, magnesium, the B vitamins and vitamin C, the two carotenes strengthen the immune system and reduce the risks of heart and arterial disease. They also cut the risks of cancer, especially of the prostate, breast, lung, colon and skin, retard the ageing process and guard the eyes against cataracts and macular degeneration and the skin against damage from UV rays.

One daily slice of pumpkin – 100–150 g (4–6 oz) – is recommended. You can roast it, make it into soup or boil and mash it with a little olive oil and black pepper.

Pumpkin seeds are very rich in omega-6 and omega-3 fatty acids (SEE *pages 12–13*), protein, minerals and vitamin E, and 5 ml (1 tsp) every other day is regarded as ample. However, they are so delicious that many people snack on them regularly or add them to muesli, rice dishes, salads, yoghurt or chopped fresh fruit.

Pure pumpkin oil, rich in essential fatty acids, magnesium, calcium and zinc, is available (SEE *Resources*).

Tomatoes

Tomatoes are high GI, but they are also very rich in lycopene, the antioxidant pigment which makes them red. Lycopene has proven anti-cancer actions: it can reduce the risks of prostate cancer by up to 35 per cent, and combat it if already established, and it helps to prevent cancers of the digestive tract. Lycopene also offers some protection against heart and arterial disease, premature ageing, dementia and other degenerative conditions.

We obtain more than 90 per cent of our lycopene from tomatoes and cooking increases its availability, so tinned tomatoes, the concentrated paste and ketchup are excellent sources. An achievable intake would be some form of cooked tomato every day and 1–2 raw tomatoes at least 5–6 days a week. Tomatoes are also rich in vitamin C, a potent antioxidant with proven anti-cancer properties, which is partly destroyed by cooking.

Protein

Protein provides amino acids, which are needed for replacing and repairing worn and damaged tissue and manufacturing hormones, enzymes and other metabolic substances. Healthy dietary protein supplies the full range of essential amino acids (those we cannot manufacture for ourselves) and is also low in saturated fat.

Especially beneficial...

Salmon
Salmon and other coldwater fish like tuna, sardines, mackerel and herring are also excellent protein sources as well as supplying fatty acids (SEE *Fats and Oils*).

Although non-organically farmed salmon has been under recent attack because it has been found to contain traces of toxins linked to birth defects and cancer, wild and organically farmed fish does not have this disadvantage. Aim to eat 1–2 100 g (4 oz) portions a week and increase this to 2–4 portions if possible.

Soya

Soya, a plant protein, comes from soya beans. It provides soluble fibre, omega-3 fatty acids (SEE *page 13*), a range of minerals and vitamins, and phytoestrogens (plant oestrogens) which can help to relieve or prevent menopausal and pre-menopausal symptoms without causing side-effects.

Soya's isoflavones – antioxidants with oestrogen-like actions – reduce the risk of several cancers, including hormone-linked breast and prostate cancer. They also offer some protection against osteoporosis, heart disease, autoimmune complaints and the deterioration of both reasoning skills and verbal and non-verbal memory. For maximum benefit, eat around 15 g (½ oz) of soya daily in two equal portions which you can obtain from tofu, soya milk, yoghurts, etc., tempeh or miso (fermented soya beans).

Turkey

Turkey is a healthy food because it has a high protein content and less saturated fat than any meat apart from liver. It is also rich in the amino acid tryptophan, needed by the brain to manufacture serotonin, a chemical mediator of mood. Low serotonin levels have been consistently found in depression sufferers and all anti-depressant drugs work to increase and preserve brain levels of serotonin and another mood chemical, noradrenaline.

Turkey also provides the trace element selenium and the B vitamin niacin, both of which have anti-cancer actions, and vitamins B6 and B12, which help to prevent heart disease. B complex vitamins are needed to release the energy from food; B12 aids the development of red blood and nerve cells and the breakdown and utilization of dietary carbohydrates, proteins and fats. You will also obtain zinc from turkey. Zinc is needed for stabilizing blood sugar levels, healing wounds and maintaining a healthy prostate gland.

The recommended intake of turkey is 100–125 mg (4–5 oz) 3–4 times weekly. If you get tired of it, add slices to stir fries or dry-fry small nuggets until crisp and eat as pre-dinner nibbles.

Fats and Oils

Fats and oils supply around 9 calories/gram as opposed to the 4 calories/gram of carbohydrates and protein. To avoid becoming overweight and to help normalize blood cholesterol, it's important to limit your total fat consumption *and* your intake of saturated fat. Hundreds of studies have linked fats from red meat and full-cream dairy products with increased risks of heart attacks, strokes, arterial disease, cancer and other disorders.

'Trans' fatty acids are also dangerous. Formed from healthy essential fatty acids during the high temperature commercial processing of plant oils, these 'anti-vitamins' have a variety of adverse effects, including interference with the production of prostaglandins, which are hormone-like substances essential for the minute-by-minute control of cellular metabolism.

However, polyunsaturates, i.e. essential fatty acids, are needed to strengthen cell membranes, facilitate the absorption of vitamins A, D and E, transport fat in the blood, regulate the menstrual cycle (through prostaglandin production), and maintain the health of the heart and arteries, skin, brain and other organs.

The older we get, the greater our need for essential fatty acids, because ageing interferes with our use of them. Weakened cell membranes are one possible reason why heart and arterial disease risks rise with age. A fatty acid shortage is also believed to be partly responsible for PMS (premenstrual syndrome), eczema-like rashes, psoriasis, allergies, autoimmune disorders, dry skin and hair, splitting nails, breast tenderness, menopausal problems, ADHD (attention deficit hyperactivity disorder), depression and possibly schizophrenia.

We obtain fatty acids from plant and fish oils. Unprocessed (cold-pressed) sunflower, safflower and corn oil (and their products, e.g. margarines) provide omega-6 linoleic acid, of which we require 5–10 g daily. (It is generally claimed that we obtain plenty from processed foods, but we are unlikely to benefit very much from them because of their conversion into the 'trans' form.) Oily fish supply omega-3 fatty acids, essential nutrients for the heart, blood vessels and brain. Green leafy vegetables also supply them, but in a precursor form (alpha-linolenic acid) which we have first to convert into the better known EPA and DHA found in fish oils (SEE *below*).

Especially beneficial...

Olive oil
Olive oil and rapeseed oil contain monounsaturated fatty acids which encourage fat-burning, cut the risks of diabetes and offer some protection against cancer and heart disease. The liberal use of olive oil in Mediterranean cooking (compared to traditional English usage) is one reason why the eponymous diet is considered so healthy. Mediterranean people, who also eat large quantities of fresh fish, fruit and vegetables, tend to be less obese than we are and have far lower risks of cardiovascular disorders. In fact, it was this observation, among others, that first prompted scientists to investigate the links between dietary fats/oils, heart attacks and strokes.

Salmon
Salmon and other oily fish such as tuna, sardines, pilchards, herring, trout and mackerel provide the omega-3 fatty acid EPA (eicosapentaenoic acid). Besides building strong cell membranes, EPA combats blood clotting, helps to lower blood pressure and increases 'good' HDL cholesterol, thereby reducing the risks of

arterial disease, heart attacks and strokes; in fact, there is evidence that eating oily fish once a week halves the risk of sudden cardiac death.

Furthermore, EPA improves bone growth and may inhibit cancer of the breast, prostate and colon – possibly explained in part by the high content of vitamin D in wild salmon. Eating salmon may also counteract some of the harmful effects of a high saturated fat intake.

Another fish oil constituent, DHA (docosahexanoic acid), EPA's close cousin, plays vital roles in brain, nerve and eye tissue. It promotes brain development in the unborn child and may reduce the chances of developing Alzheimer's disease, other dementias and the age-related deterioration of reasoning and memory.

Aim to eat 1–2 100 g (4 oz) portions a week and increase this to 2–4 portions if possible. If you hate fish, take an odourless fish oil supplement instead.

Walnuts

Walnuts, with their 7:1 ratio of polyunsaturated to saturated fat, cholesterol-reducing plant serums and omega-3 oils, have the highest antioxidant action of all nuts, followed by almonds and pistachios. They are a high-energy food, but should be enjoyed regularly – a handful 4–5 times weekly can significantly lower your blood cholesterol *and* can reduce your risks of suffering a heart attack by between 15 and 51 per cent.

2

Herbal Medicine

MEDICINAL PLANTS SUCH as the opium poppy, mandrake, belladonna, rhubarb and quince were mentioned by Hippocrates as long ago as 420 BC, when he classified herbs and foods as hot, cold, dry and damp to correspond with man's four humours – black and yellow bile, blood and phlegm. Galen, personal physician to the philosopher Marcus Aurelius, elaborated upon this in the second century AD, placing many foods into more than one category according to their effects upon the humours. Cold, moist foods such as beans, for example, were believed to increase phlegm, so eating too many could cause catarrh. On the other hand, too many hot dry foods such as millet, onions and mustard seed produced excessive quantities of yellow bile and could harm the skin or liver.

Our habit of discriminating between plant foods and herbs is largely a product of the nineteenth and twentieth centuries. In the seventeenth century, carrots, cabbage, cucumbers and other common foods were classified as herbs, and medieval recipes reveal how foods tended to be cooked and served with their balancing counterparts. 'Damp' barley and oatmeal both went well with 'dry' honey, and 'cold' lettuce was suitably partnered by 'hot' onions.

This emphasis upon harmony is reflected today in the preparation of herbal remedies from whole plants which medical herbalists recognize as balanced, living organisms. Preparing medicines from them in their natural state provides a valuable buffering against possible side-effects, and synergistic action between constituents, which enhances the desired effects.

The dandelion is a good example. Its leaves act as a gentle but effective diuretic, boosting urine flow, at the same time supplying potassium to make good its loss in the increased urine output. In fact, this plant achieves naturally what pharmaceutical scientists have spent millions of pounds trying to emulate. Thiazide diuretics and furosemide, routinely prescribed for patients with high blood pressure and cardiac problems, cause potassium loss which, if excessive, can interfere with the heart's rhythm and trigger cardiac arrest. Supplementary potassium is prescribed, although it is frequently not taken because many patients are unaware of why they need it. Sometimes 'potassium sparing' diuretics are prescribed instead, but they are often less effective than the more established furosemide and thiazides.

Herbal Holism

Many herbal remedies are selected like prescribed drugs to relieve symptoms. You might take feverfew for migraine instead of paracetamol or nurofen, for example, or ginger to relieve motion sickness. However, this approach flies in the face of tradition. Like all holistic therapies, 'real' herbal medicine addresses the underlying imbalances rather than the symptoms. Over-the-counter herbal remedies bring relief, but medical herbalists work at a deeper level to improve vitality and physical and psychological balance.

Herbal practitioners, like orthodox doctors, take a case history, but include questions about stress, inherited complaints, emotional well-being, exercise, diet and relaxation. Their examination and diagnostic aids may be similarly orthodox, but they may also include holistic tests such as pulse examination (a feature of acupuncture) or iridology (examination of the irises). Herbal doctors also tend to word their diagnosis in terms of the underlying 'disease' process rather than labelling the complaint. You might be told that you are suffering from eye inflammation, for instance, instead of bacterial conjunctivitis, or bowel spasm rather than irritable bowel syndrome.

The aim of herbal medicine is to enhance the body's inherent self-healing capabilities. Treatment is prescribed according to the aspect of health most in need of adjustment and the herbs are chosen for an appropriate mode of action, which can be challenging, directing or eliminating.

Challenging

Challenging herbs provoke protective responses from the body. Examples include senna, which stimulates bowel movement and relieves constipation, and diuretics such as dandelion, corn silk and couch grass, which stimulate urine flow.

Body-process directing

These herbs bring about the desired effects in body tissues and organs. Examples include hawthorn preparations, which increase coronary artery blood flow and slow the pulse rate (useful in cases of heart failure), and Korean ginseng, which has a tonic effect upon the adrenal glands and thereby on the body's response to stress.

Eliminatory

These herbs encourage one or more of the body's eliminatory functions and are used to speed up the removal of metabolites and toxins. Examples include diuretics (SEE *page 17*), expectorants to help bring up phlegm from the chest, e.g. heartsease, cowslip, balm of Gilead and white horehound, and emetics which induce vomiting, e.g. ipecacuanha, lobelia, squills and snake root.

Common Herbal Remedies

Most people perceive herbal remedies as safe, gentle and free from side-effects. Generally speaking, this is true, but substances powerful enough to relieve pain, nausea and diarrhoea, and, in their prescribed form, treat heart disease and cancer, clearly have the potential for harm if misused.

The action of too much senna on a constipated bowel, for example, is anything but gentle. The over-generous use of nutmeg for nausea, vomiting and indigestion is decidedly unsafe and can cause terrifying nightmares and hallucinations, while a single 7½ g dose can trigger palpitations and convulsions. Many herbal remedies can be toxic, even lethal, in large amounts and, like conventional drugs, you need to take them exactly as directed.

> **CAUTION:** Check with your doctor before taking herbal remedies if you are receiving treatment for a medical condition. Treat simple ailments only and seek medical or qualified herbal advice for more major problems, in cases where you are unsure of the diagnosis, or where simple treatments fail to help. Never use any herbal preparation when pregnant unless prescribed by a qualified medical practitioner.

Aloe vera

Aloe vera is taken internally as a digestive aid and to ease painful heartburn and gastritis. The gel and liquid are also useful for minor burns, including sunburn, bites and stings, dermatitis, eczema and athlete's foot.

Calendula

Good for inflamed skin, sores, bruises and minor rashes, calendula is also used as a wash, cream and tincture, and sometimes prescribed as an infusion (SEE *page 24*) for mumps, swollen glands, tonsillitis and childhood fevers.

Chamomile

A popular sedative herbal remedy, chamomile tea is drunk to overcome insomnia and to aid digestion. The cream or lotion soothes inflamed skin conditions.

Cinnamon

A warming remedy for colds, coughs and fevers, cinnamon is also prescribed for rheumatic complaints and is a handy kitchen remedy for nausea, vomiting and diarrhoea (stir a large pinch into water or milk just off the boil, let stand for a minute or two and sip slowly).

Comfrey

Also known as knit-bone, comfrey ointment or cream has been used for centuries to relieve arthritis, sprains and strains, and to help unite fractures. It is also prescribed for certain gastric complaints, and for eczema and psoriasis.

Dandelion

Dandelion is prescribed to boost liver and kidney function. The leaves are rich in vitamin A and potassium and are pleasant in a salad. The milky juice from the cut stem gets rid of warts and verrucae.

Echinacea

Widely used to boost immunity against bacterial, viral and fungal infections, echinacea is also useful for tonsillitis, mouth and tongue infections, abscesses and boils, and as a mouthwash for sore gums.

Fennel

Tea made from fennel seeds relieves flatulence (wind) and colic. Some breastfeeding mothers take it to promote their milk flow and prevent infant colic. It is also a useful eyewash for sore eyes.

Feverfew

This is a widely used remedy for the relief of migraines, other forms of headache and painful periods. Many migraine sufferers grow feverfew and make a sandwich of the freshly picked leaves when an attack threatens. It can also help to relieve rheumatic disorders and arthritis.

Garlic

Garlic has powerful antiseptic properties and can offer protection against bacterial, fungal and viral infections, including intestinal and chest infections, colds and flu. It has numerous beneficial actions on the heart and circulation, helping to reduce high blood pressure and to normalize total cholesterol, reducing levels of harmful LDL cholesterol and elevating levels of the protective HDL variety.

Garlic acts as a vasodilator, relaxing constricted blood vessels, and counteracts the blood's clotting actions. It encourages wound healing and reduces the pain and inflammation of insect bites and stings. In addition, it helps to stabilize the blood sugar level. When used in a specially prepared oil, it soothes middle ear congestion and inflammation and combats the infection, encouraging the healing process.

Ginkgo biloba

Extracts of the fresh leaves of ginkgo biloba (usually as tablets or capsules) have been marketed in Europe for decades for the treatment of arterial disease of the brain (dementia and Alzheimer's disease, age-related cognitive decline) and for disorders of the peripheral circulation (including piles, varicose veins and leg ulcers). Research has also confirmed that the leaves' constituents, chemicals called ginkgolides, can work as effectively as standard prescription drugs to relieve severely irregular heart rhythms.

Ginseng (Korean, Asiatic)

Ginseng is an adaptogen, meaning that it improves the overall balance of bodily functions. It has beneficial effects upon the adrenal cortex and hypothalamus (a master gland in the brain), both of which help us deal more effectively with stress. It also relaxes and stimulates parts of the central nervous system, improves muscular stamina and helps to combat high blood sugar levels, with beneficial effects upon the heart and liver.

Ginseng (Siberian)

Also an adaptogen, Siberian ginseng is substantially similar to Korean ginseng but has more of a stimulant action. Taken to improve stamina in face of excessive mental, emotional and physical demands, it also increases resistance to disease, infections, age-related changes and cold climates. One claimed effect is the reversal of arterial disease in its early stages. It may be helpful for diabetes and certain heart problems.

Lemon balm

Also called melissa and bee balm, lemon balm gently encourages perspiration and can be used to ease colds, flu and other feverish ailments. As a pleasant-tasting slightly sedative tea, it is suitable for bedtime drinks.

Marshmallow

Marshmallow soothes inflamed membranes lining the digestive, urinary and respiratory tracts, so is prescribed for bronchitis, cystitis and stomach/bowel irritations. Infusions are sometimes used to relieve dry skin.

Nettle

Nettle has tonic, astringent and diuretic properties, and is prescribed/used as a blood tonic and cleanser and as a source of iron. You can infuse fresh nettles to make a drink or cook them like spinach (don't inhale the steam, which contains the formic acid responsible for their sting). Add a boiled potato or two to cooked nettles to dilute the strong flavour before blending into a soup or purée. Nettles are also useful for hair and scalp complaints, and extracts are often added to shampoo and other hair products.

Peppermint

Refreshing and cleansing, peppermint tea relieves colic, wind, indigestion, nausea and headaches linked with indigestion. It can also help period pain. The cool infusion soothes hot itchy skin conditions.

Raspberry

Teas containing the fruit taste good and supply vitamin C, which boosts immunity. Raspberry leaf tea is often prescribed during the last stages of pregnancy and during labour to facilitate delivery.

Rosemary

Rosemary has anti-inflammatory and tonic properties. An infusion can relieve headaches and a low mood, colds and colic. Rosemary also relieves dandruff and the ancient Greeks tucked sprigs of it behind their ears prior to sitting examinations, as a valuable memory aid.

Slippery elm

Slippery elm soothes inflamed mucous membranes of the digestive tract, which is useful after an attack of gastroenteritis or when suffering from a peptic ulcer.

St John's wort (Hypericum)

Widely taken to relieve mild to moderate depression, allay anxiety and encourage sound sleep, St John's wort is also an excellent wound healer and comes as a cream in combination with calendula extract under the brand name Hypercal for minor cuts and abrasions.

Thyme

A useful antiseptic and expectorant remedy for colds, coughs and chest infections, thyme is also a soothing remedy for irritable bowel and upset stomach. Medical herbalists prescribe it for urinary tract infections.

Valerian

Widely used to relieve insomnia and nervous tension, valerian is gently tranquillizing without being addictive. Its common name, heal-all, refers to its wide range of therapeutic properties: applied locally to painful tissue areas, it relieves muscular cramp and stiffness, has a gently 'warming' effect on 'cold' conditions such as rheumatism and osteoarthritis, and acts as a diuretic (increasing urine flow) and an expectorant (helping to clear mucus from upper airways and lungs).

Preparing Herbs

> **CAUTION:** If mixing herbs, the total amount should not exceed the quantities mentioned for single herb use.

Infusion

This is the simplest way of using many herbs. An infusion is made like a tea, utilizing the tender parts like flowers and leaves.

Standard quantities: 75 g (3 oz) fresh or 30 g (1 oz) dried herb to 500 ml (1 pint) water.

Method: Pour water just off the boil onto the herb, leave to infuse for up to ten minutes, strain and drink/use hot or cold. Make fresh daily.

Standard dose: one teacup or wineglassful three times daily.

Useful for chamomile, peppermint, rosemary.

Decoction

This is a more energetic extraction method, used for roots, bark, firm berries and seeds.

Standard quantities: 60 g (2 oz) fresh or 30 g (1 oz) dried herb to 750 ml (1½ pints) water reduced to 500 ml (1 pint) with heating.

Method: Heat the herb in cold water and simmer for up to 1 hour. Strain, drink/use hot or cold. Make fresh daily.

Standard dose: one teacup or wineglassful three times daily.

Useful for ginger, rosehips, ginseng.

Steam inhalant

Method: Place 15–30 ml (1–2 tbsp) of the dried herb in a basin and pour boiling water over it. Lean over the bowl with a towel over your head and the bowl, and inhale for as long as you can, or until the preparation cools.

Used to treat sinusitis and other airways infections.

Compress

This is a cloth soaked in a herbal extract, e.g. a standard infusion, and applied either hot or cold to the affected area.

Cold compresses relieve headaches. A lavender compress, for example, can be made utilizing the cool infusion or 3–4 drops of essential oil added to cold water (SEE *Aromatherapy*).

Hot compresses relieve muscular pain and encourage wound healing. Use a standard infusion or a 5–20 ml tincture (which you can purchase) in 500 ml (1 pint) of hot water. An angelica hot compress, for example, can be used to treat rheumatic pain and osteoarthritis.

Poultice

A poultice is like a compress, but nearly always applied hot and utilizes the whole herb rather than the extract.

Method: Boil the fresh herb in a little water for 5 minutes, using enough to cover the area. Cool slightly and squeeze out the surplus liquid. Use it to moisten the skin to prevent sticking, then bind the herb in place with a cloth or bandage.

You can also make the powdered herb or its crushed seeds into a paste with water.

Suitable for powdered fenugreek, to relieve *boils* and cellulitis (soft tissue inflammation), and for fresh coltsfoot leaves to encourage healing in slow-to-respond skin lesions such as ulcers and sores.

Bach Flower Remedies

This plant-derived therapy was devised during the late 1920s and 1930s by Dr Edward Bach, a physician, homoeopath and bacteriologist. He recognized the huge role played in disease by stress and negative emotions, something we are becoming increasingly aware of today.

While treating his patients, Dr Bach observed that people with different complaints but similar outlook and personalities often responded to the same remedy. Conversely, patients with the same disorder who differed temperamentally and emotionally generally needed different remedies. Early on, he formulated the axiom: 'Take no notice of the disease, think only of the personality of the one in distress.' Like Samuel Hahnemann before him (SEE *Homoeopathy*), he found many of the extant medical treatments too harsh and he left a lucrative London practice to return home to north Wales in search of a new healing system lacking side-effects.

The flower remedies and holism

While Bach believed that the use of poisonous animal, plant and mineral substances to be bad medicine, even in infinitesimal quantities, he was aware from his homoeopathic training that extremely dilute substances can stimulate the body's self-healing powers. A born healer and a 'sensitive', he was convinced that particular wild plants held the secret to genuine cures. He was, in fact, so closely attuned to their vibrational qualities (the existence of which has since been established by quantum physicists), that he could detect the likely benefits of a flowering plant on body, mind and spirit simply by holding his hands over it or placing a single petal on his tongue.

Dr Bach deduced that certain flowers were of a higher order, with greater therapeutic potential, than ordinary medicinal plants that heal at a grosser level. He believed that true plant healers rectify imbalances within the psychological and spiritual spheres, changing such negative emotions as panic, distrust of self, hopelessness and excessive submissiveness into their life-affirming opposites – courage, self-confidence, renewed hope and constructive self-assertiveness. Thus Bach treated the whole person, correcting inner conflict and negativity and bringing relief and healing.

The Remedies

Edward Bach identified seven negative emotional states which he broke down into thirty-eight negative emotions, each linked to a particular plant. He made up his flower remedies by floating fresh blooms on the surface of bowls of fresh pure water from a rocky stream near his home and leaving them to be irradiated by sunlight. The water, he believed, picked up the plants' vibrational essence, much as the repeated succussion (mechanical agitation) employed in homoeopathy imbues the solvent with the medicinal substance's imprint. Bach's vitalized liquid, carefully strained through twigs from the remedy plant to avoid contamination, then became the remedy's stock.

Next, Bach added an equal volume of brandy to form his 'mother tincture'; this in turn was further diluted with brandy. The resulting liquid, the stock concentrate, was the form in which the remedies were used.

There are 39 Bach Flower Remedies – 37 from individual wild flowers, one from Rock Water (pure water from a rocky stream) and the well-known Rescue Remedy, based on Cherry Plum, Clematis, Impatiens, Star of Bethlehem and Rock Rose, to treat humans and animals who are injured or shocked. The Remedies' full mode of action is incompletely understood, but their usefulness is reflected by their popularity, the response of animals to the Rescue Remedy, and the relief gained by babies and small children.

Examples include:

Chicory: For a demanding nature, self-pity, self-love; possessive, hurt and tearful feelings

Gentian: For discouragement, melancholy, doubt

Gorse: For lack of hope, the acceptance of chronic illness or difficulty, the feeling that it is pointless to try

Red Chestnut: For worry for others, anticipating misfortune, for projecting anxiety into trusting to life

Rock Water: For self-denial, a rigid outlook, purist tendencies

3

Aromatherapy

AROMATHERAPY IS THE treatment of ailments and diseases with aromatic pure plant essences. Its name is a product of the twentieth century but, like herbal medicine, its origins can be traced back to ancient times. Egyptian papyri dating from 2890 BC record the medicinal use of aniseed, cedar, cumin, coriander and other aromatic plants, including their smoke and ashes. Clay tablets record that the infused oils of cedar and cypress were imported into Egypt, and traces of styrax, frankincense and other aromatics have been identified in ointment and cosmetic jars found in the pyramids.

The ancient Greeks, who acquired some of their medical knowledge from the Egyptians, used olive oil saturated with plant perfumes for culinary, cosmetic, religious and medicinal purposes, and made ointments of myrrh to treat wounds.

After the fall of Rome, the hub of medical knowledge switched to the Byzantine empire, and the Arab physician Avicenna (AD 980–1037) left written records of more than 800 medicinal plants, including the aromatics chamomile, camphor and lavender – three of the most widely used essential oils in present times. Most importantly, he is said to have discovered the process of steam distillation still used today to extract pure essences. Many of these aromatic records, together with the secrets of distillation, reached Europe during the early Middle Ages and physicians were soon distilling a range of essences including lavender, thyme and rosemary.

Aromatic plants and their extracts continued to feature in traditional medical practice in Europe and the Middle East, India and China, and interest in the oils became more widespread in the 1920s with the discoveries of René Maurice Gattefossé. A chemist in his family's perfume company in France, Gattefossé observed the non-toxic antiseptic properties of the essential oils and suggested their use in perfume-making in preference to harsh synthetic chemicals. Responsible for the modern term 'aromatherapy', Gattefossé went on to develop the use of essential oils to treat skin diseases after neat lavender oil healed his badly burned hand swiftly and without scarring.

Holistic Aromatherapy

Today aromatherapy is one of the most popular complementary therapies. The oils are easy to carry around, can relieve a wide range of symptoms and ailments, and are entirely safe if used according to directions. Treatment is pleasant, effective and relatively inexpensive. Essential oils are available from high street pharmacies, health food stores and other outlets, and professional treatment can be obtained from holistic therapy centres, Yellow Pages and/or personal recommendation.

Qualified aromatherapists, who may practise other therapies or specialize in aromatherapy, look beyond the relief of symptoms to their underlying cause. Most seek information about an ailment's origin, the factors that aggravate or relieve it, the person's general health and susceptibility to other complaints, including infections. They are also interested in a person's diet, activity level, responses to stress and patterns of sleep, rest and relaxation. The aim of the questions, as with any holistic therapy, is to identify physical, psychological or emotional imbalance.

Essential oils work holistically at several different levels. Extracted from whole plants (as opposed to the isolated active constituents of pharmaceuticals), they contain natural ingredients which counterbalance each other's actions and work simultaneously on body, mind and spirit.

Lavender oil, for example, contains ethers of linalyl and geranyl, geraniol, linalol, cineol, d-borneol, limonene, 1-pinene, caryophyllene, butyric acid and valerianic acid esters, and coumarin. The ratio of its various ingredients – and therefore, to an extent, its effects – varies from region to region, reflecting the soil quality, other growing conditions and climate. This helps to explain lavender oil's spectrum of actions, which includes pain relief, raising a low mood, soothing anxiety and tension, killing bacteria, relieving congestion, reducing high blood pressure, repelling insects and getting rid of intestinal worms. Its greatest asset is its balancing effect on the body and mind, a vital prerequisite for holistic healing. A remedy's spiritual benefits are hard to define, but most of us who have inhaled lavender essence when miserable, sleepless or fraught have experienced the reassuring sense of calm that makes it such a favourite.

Using Aromatherapy Oils

Essential oil molecules pass through the skin into the bloodstream and thence around the body. Massage is generally used to administer the oils professionally and there is no doubt that physical contact with the practitioner, combined with their empathy and willingness to listen, plays an important healing role. You can benefit from the 'touch' aspect when using the oils at home either by enlisting the help of your partner or a family member or by using a simple massage technique on yourself.

Massage

For massage purposes, you need to dilute aromatherapy oils with a carrier oil because most are too strong to be placed directly upon the skin; the carrier solvent also provides the necessary lubrication. Cold-pressed additive-free vegetable oils such as sunflower or soya are good choices, as are sweet almond and grapeseed oil. Olive oil is unsuitable because its odour interferes with the aroma (although it could be used if there were no alternative). More specialist oils with a high nutrient content like macadamia nut and avocado also feed dry delicate skin. Some people use vitamin E-rich wheatgerm oil because it helps to prevent scar formation and the signs of ageing, but it is too viscous for effective lubrication and is usually added to sunflower or some other carrier oil in the proportion of 1:4.

It's a sound idea to estimate how much massage oil you are going to need and make it up fresh each time to prevent the oils turning rancid. Label directions may offer a guide to the quantities of essential oil to be used, but a reliable rule of thumb is to add 3 drops of essential oil to 5 ml (1 tsp) carrier oil. Depending on the area of skin to be treated, you could start by mixing 6 drops of essential oil with 10 ml (2 tsp) carrier oil, and see how you make out.

For a shared relaxation massage, rose is a popular choice because of its aphrodisiac properties. It is especially attuned to women's needs, including the improvement of unsatisfactory body image and confidence levels. Sandalwood can increase sexual desire in men and women (though men seem especially fond of it), neroli works well for both, and jasmine encourages a light-hearted, positive and confident attitude to love-making, especially in men.

CAUTION: Massage can be harmful in some circumstances. Do not massage over injuries or broken skin, varicose veins or recent scar tissue. Avoid massage during pregnancy and if suffering from an inflammatory condition, thrombosis, heart disease or other serious disorder. Massage should also be avoided straight after a meal or drinking session, where there is a high temperature or acute infection, and for ten days following vaccination. If in doubt, consult your doctor or medical adviser.

Never take essential oils by mouth except under the guidance of a medically qualified practitioner.

Inhalation

Nerve cells in the lining of the nose responsible for the sense of smell link directly through tiny holes in the skull with the frontal lobes of the brain. Stimulation of these cells by aromatic substances quickly reaches the brain, which also receives any active constituents passing into the bloodstream through the airways' lining membranes and/or the skin. This helps to explain the rapid relief to be gained from a variety of ailments by inhalation of essential oils, either from a few drops on a tissue tucked under your pillow or in your upper pocket, or added to steaming hot water.

The towel-over-head inhalation method (SEE *page 151*), is particularly effective for catarrh and other ailments of the upper airways. The warm steam itself dilutes and softens thick phlegm, and lavender, tea tree, rosemary, thyme and eucalyptus are appropriate choices of oil.

You can also enjoy the perfume of your favourite oils by adding a few drops of them to a carrier oil and warming the mixture in a specially designed burner. Some of the better (more costly) candles on the market contain genuine aromatherapy essences and are useful aids to relaxation and meditation.

Aromatherapy baths

There are many aroma-related products on the market for enhancing the therapeutic effects of baths and showers.

To help you unwind and relax, look for bath oils and shower gels containing genuine essence of bergamot, lavender or chamomile, among others, or add a few drops of the oil(s) to the bathwater.

To combat morning exhaustion and boost your alertness and vitality, have a stimulating cold shower or bath and use essences of thyme, grapefruit, rosemary, lavender or peppermint.

Aromatherapy Essences

The following oils are widely used and readily available; only a selection of their beneficial effects has been included.

Clary sage

Clary sage has an uplifting effect because it relieves anxiety and tension. It can be used to help lift depression and a clary sage massage after a relaxing bath can induce both euphoria and sound sleep. It also helps to relieve an itchy scalp, inflamed skin and rheumatic or muscular aches and pains.

> **CAUTION:** Never use clary sage in any form after you have been drinking. Even a low alcohol concentration in the blood can combine with the oil's active constituents to produce appalling nightmares.

Eucalyptus

Eucalyptus is an excellent antiseptic and decongestant with power-ful anti-bacterial and anti-viral actions. When inhaled in steam, it reduces nasal stuffiness due to catarrh and helps to prevent colds and flu. Used with essence of bergamot, it helps to clear up herpes simplex (cold) sores. It also promotes healing by keeping infection at bay and enhancing new cell growth.

Frankincense

The perfume of this powerfully aromatic resinous oil induces states of near-ecstasy in some people. It makes a good inhalation for asthma because it soothes the inflamed airways and calms panic. Frankincense is also included in beauty preparations for ageing skin.

Geranium

Geranium has a delightful mint/rose perfume and is widely used in skin care. It relieves a range of complaints from acne, bruises and cellulite to menopausal problems, nervous tension and pre-menstrual syndrome. It also repels mosquitoes.

Ginger

Ginger is warming and drying (SEE *Herbal Medicine*), and it reduces phlegm and catarrh and combats nausea and vomiting. It relieves arthritis and muscular pain (though consult a medical practitioner before using it for an arthritis rub when the disease is active).

Grapefruit

This oil clears the mind and lifts the spirits and is mainly used as a mental and physical tonic. It counteracts jet lag and travel fatigue generally, stimulates the digestive and lymphatic systems and combats oily skin.

Jasmine

The forte of this luxurious, wonderfully perfumed oil is its skin-balancing action. Widely used in perfumes and cosmetics, it soothes dry skin conditions. Inhaling a couple of drops of jasmine essence or adding them to bathwater lifts stress, exhaustion and PMS symptoms, as well as general aches and pains. You will feel more cheerful and relaxed after its use.

Juniper

Refreshing and cleansing, juniper essential oil combats water retention and can reduce the discomfort of cystitis. A juniper bath or inhalation has a tonic effect upon body and mind. Qualified aromatherapists use this oil to treat gout and some types of rheumatism.

Lavender

Lavender has an incomparably comforting and uplifting action upon a tense, anxious mind and tired body. It is one of the few oils which can safely be used neat on the skin – a drop or two rubbed onto the temples helps to relieve migraine attacks and other headaches. It soothes and promotes the healing of grazes, cuts and skin injuries, minor burns and sunburn. Essence of lavender is also used to treat eczema, fungal infections and a flaking scalp.

Lemon

Antiseptic and refreshing, lemon essential oil can combat infectious diseases, especially feverish colds. It's a circulatory aid and can relieve migraine and tension headaches. It is also a tonic for oily skin and may help to combat nausea.

Mandarin

A cheerful, gentle essential oil, mandarin stimulates the digestion and helps to restore the appetite following an illness. It tends to be popular with children and it both revives and strengthens a positive outlook.

Neroli

An oil from the flowers of the bitter orange, neroli is soothing and uplifting. It is useful in cases of PMS, severe anxiety and other emotional problems, and combats nervous dyspepsia. It is widely used in the cosmetic and perfume industries.

Peppermint

A refreshing clean-scented essential oil useful in relieving bowel spasm (colic and others), wind and other digestive problems. It clears the head of nasal stuffiness and can help cure fatigue, throbbing headaches and migraine.

Roman Chamomile

A very soothing, warming and calming oil for rashes and insect bites, joint and muscle pain, indigestion and all types of headache including migraine.

Rose

Richly floral and feminine, rose oil is excellent for female problems. It helps to regulate irregular periods and combats loss of interest in love-making (especially when linked to recent weight gain and/or the menopause). Its aphrodisiac properties work especially well for women with poor sexual confidence and self-esteem.

Rosemary

An invigorating oil which revives the body and mind when stressed and fatigued, rosemary is used in massage to relieve stiff painful muscles and period pain. Inhaling it relieves headaches and helps to clear nasal stuffiness and blocked sinuses.

Sandalwood

Comforting and relaxing, sandalwood relieves dry coughs and dry skin conditions such as eczema and psoriasis. It can also be useful in cases of diarrhoea and cystitis.

Tea tree

Powerfully antiseptic and anti-fungal, tea tree oil, which can also be used neat, is one of the most widely used essences. It helps to clear up cold sores, vaginal thrush, athlete's foot, boils and wound infections, cystitis and various infectious illnesses.

Yarrow

Yarrow is a balancing and healing oil of benefit for most inflammatory skin disorders, and for indigestion and wind. Therapists use it for its restorative and psychologically strengthening effects.

Ylang ylang

Ylang ylang has an emotionally balancing effect upon highly strung individuals and anyone in crisis. It can have a powerfully sedative effect and is often used to treat insomnia. It has a delight-ful scent similar to hyacinths in spring and, like lavender essential oil, a quick sniff of the neat oil brings comfort and tranquillity when most needed. Ylang ylang is often found in skincare prod-ucts, cosmetics and floral perfumes.

4

Homoeopathy

M ANY OF US turn to homoeopathic remedies to relieve minor ailments, but they are less simple than they at first appear – to work most effectively, they have to suit both the illness and the person taking them. Understanding a little more about this can help you to choose the right treatment. The remedies for self-treatment are widely available from pharmacies, health stores, mail order companies and internet sites. Also consider consulting a qualified practitioner should you need to do so.

Homoeopathy was first practised in Britain in 1832 after a Dr Hervey Quin, who had studied the treatment in Leipzig, returned to London and set up practice. Homoeopathy had been used in Germany since the second half of the eighteenth century following its discovery by a physician, Dr Samuel Hahnemann. Quin became the first president of the British Homoeopathic Society when it was founded in 1844 and since then, despite opposition from many establishment doctors, homoeopathic medicine has grown ever more popular.

At the start of the twenty-first century, there are five homoeopathic hospitals in Britain where patients receive both homoeopathic and conventional medical treatment. More than 1,000 GPs and hospital doctors are members of the Faculty of Homoeopathy, alongside many non-medically qualified practitioners. The Queen uses homoeopathy and has her own specially appointed homoeopathic physician. Homoeopathic consultations are available on the NHS and homoeopathic remedies can be prescribed on ordinary EC10 prescription forms.

The chief attractions of homoeopathy are its effectiveness, its safety, its accessibility, its usefulness for many conditions and its suitability for people of all ages, from the newborn to the very elderly. With so many points in its favour, why does it remain controversial? A major stumbling block to its universal acceptance is our incomplete understanding of how it works.

During a consultation, homoeopathic practitioners (homoeopaths), like orthodox doctors, take their patient's medical history and carry out an examination and tests. Both orthodox and homoeopathic medicine ultimately depend upon the body's inherent self-regulating, self-healing mechanism for a cure. But here the differences become more apparent. If you visited your GP complaining of painful swollen joints, for instance, they might diagnose osteoarthritis, recommend gentle exercise, weight loss and physiotherapy, and prescribe an anti-inflammatory drug such as ibuprofen or nurofen. A homoeopath would ask many more questions. They would want an account of your medical history from pre-birth onwards, plus details of your appetite, bowel function, personal tastes, diet, exercise and lifestyle, and any factors aggravating or relieving your symptoms. They would also need to know about your emotional state and how you function at work (if applicable), at home and in your relationships. They would be looking for the causes of the imbalances triggering your condition and for clues to the remedy likeliest to help.

Importantly, because homoeopathy is naturopathic (i.e. it works with nature to promote healing), the homoeopath would also suggest appropriate lifestyle changes. The wrong diet, too little or too much exercise, smoking and heavy drinking, poor stress control and emotional wear and tear all weaken the subtle 'Vital Force' regarded from the homoeopathic standpoint as the lynchpin of health. Then, based on the picture they had formed of your disorder, your personality, your constitutional type and other factors, the homoeopath would prescribe a remedy, which they would dispense themselves or which you could obtain from a homoeopathic pharmacist.

Obviously, the allopathic (conventional) concept of disease differs radically from the homoeopathic model. Orthodox practitioners regard the stiff joint, the sore throat, the stomachache and vomiting, for example, as evidence of arthritis, an infection or a stomach upset – diseases *per se* which they set out to cure with drugs that antagonize and damp down the symptoms. Homoeopaths interpret symptoms as the body's efforts to restore balance and health. Instead of suppressing them, they encourage the body's attempts to heal itself with remedies which evoke the same symptoms.

Nux vomica, for example, which in non-homoeopathic doses causes vomiting, is often used to relieve nausea, sickness and hangovers. Apis mellifica, derived from whole bees and/or their venom, is useful for insect bites, the stinging, burning rashes of infectious illnesses such as chickenpox and shingles, and for allergic reactions.

In his book *The Family Guide to Homoeopathy: The Safe Form of Medicine for the Future*, Dr Andrew Lockie offers a brilliant illustration of the rationale behind this approach. He likens the Vital Force to a trampoline and the stresses which we all encounter to stones dropped on it randomly from a great height. If the Vital Force is flowing strongly, the trampoline, being taut, will fling off even biggish stones. But if it is weak and dissipated, the trampoline will sag. It will lack the recoil energy to fling the stones off, so some will settle, making it sag even more. The only way to trigger a recoil strong enough to leave it stone-free is to bounce something much heavier on the trampoline in the hope that the recoil will be powerful enough to throw off the accumulating stones together with the heavy object. 'This, essentially, is what homoeopathic remedies do in cases of chronic illness,' says Dr Lockie. 'They are the stimuli which energise the Vital Force.'

'Like May Be Cured by Like...'

Homoeopathy developed from Samuel Hahnemann's experiments with cinchona bark extract (quinine), used to treat swamp fever (malaria). So many of the medical practices of his day were, in his opinion, barbaric that he was eager to discover alternative treatments. Wondering why the astringent quinine should work for malaria when stronger astringents did not, he took some himself and noted, to his surprise, that it gave him malaria-like symptoms – high fever, perspiration, rigors (violent shaking) and profound weakness. If these ills were produced by a curative medicine, Hahnemann reflected, could the symptoms of malaria possibly represent the body's attempts to shake the illness off?

Hahnemann then proceeded to test first quinine then other substances such as sulphur, arsenic and mercury on friends and acquaintances who had to be both physically and mentally fit *and* willing to forgo highly spiced foods, alcohol, coffee, tea and 'all disturbing passions' in case they interfered with the results. These initial tests, or 'provings', as Hahnemann called them, produced a whole host of symptoms in the volunteers, varying in both type and intensity from one individual to another. Common or 'first-line' symptoms, less common or 'second-line' symptoms and 'third-line' rare or idiosyncratic symptoms were noted for each substance.

Having built up a 'drug picture' in this way for a wide range of medicines, Hahnemann then proceeded to try them out on patients. First he built up a profile of the individual he proposed to treat, based on their complaint and how their symptoms were affected by their emotions, time of day, weather, environment and other factors; a physical examination, general health and lifestyle, attitudes, moods and psychological health. He then matched this 'symptom picture' with the 'drug picture' it most resembled.

The closer the fit, Hahnemann found, the more effective the remedy: in some way, a remedy and a disease that produced the same symptoms cancelled one another out. The truth of the adage 'Like may be cured by like' had been borne out by this newly discovered medical system.

Further developments followed when Hahnemann discovered that some of his patients became worse before starting to recover. He began diluting his medicines, leaving a particular substance, for example a plant or mineral fragment, to stand in alcohol for a month, then carefully pouring off the liquid and diluting a single drop of this 'mother tincture' with 99 drops of alcohol. This 1:100 dilution, or first centesimal potency, was designated 1c. Successive dilutions, each by a factor of 100, produced further centesimal potencies of 2c, 3c and so on.

Hahnemann mixed each dilution extremely thoroughly by a process called 'succussion' which involved their being banged on a hard surface for a specific length of time. To his surprise, he discovered that this not only banished the unpleasant side-effects, but also brought faster, more effective relief. *In fact, the greater a remedy's dilution, the more powerful its effect.*

This 'potentization' of medicines by repeated dilution was a paradox which Hahnemann could never entirely explain, especially since, by the eleventh or twelfth dilution (11c and 12c), it was doubtful whether a single molecule of the original substance remained. He surmised, however, that his remedies were influencing some sort of subtle energy or Vital Force which normally kept body and mind functioning harmoniously and protected them from disease. When it was upset by stress, poor nutrition, inherited weaknesses or climatic change, illness resulted; the body then fought to restore its equilibrium, i.e. health, giving rise to symptoms in the process.

It is now believed that the vigorous succussion leaves an impression of the active substance's energy blueprint on the molecules of solvent. This may indeed be so, since quantum physics has recently discovered that material matter is not actually solid, but instead consists of electromagnetic energy; the material objects that we perceive as 'hard' and 'solid' are actually comprised of wavelengths, each with its own vibrational pattern.

In the case of chronic or long-standing complaints with relapses and remissions, for example rheumatoid arthritis or peptic ulcer, the Vital Force has to strive continually against ongoing adverse factors and needs carefully prescribed specific remedies – in other words, the 'heavy weight dropped from a height' mentioned in Dr Lockie's trampoline analogy. In the case of acute ailments, for example the common cold, headache or upset stomach, which come on suddenly, produce familiar symptoms then go away again after a while, the Vital Force remains comparatively strong and the remedies affect it more as a catalyst or 'helping hand'.

Treating Yourself

Self-treatment with homoeopathic remedies is a less sophisticated procedure than homoeopathic prescribing, which takes into account such features as 'miasms' (underlying health problems, e.g. viral infections and depression, which cause intermittent outbreaks of illness) and 'constitutional types' (categories into which individuals fall according to key characteristics, including their reaction to certain remedies). But while the same remedy will suit most people suffering from common disorders such as hayfever, a cold or toothache, individual symptoms remain important and should be considered wherever feasible.

If you want to refine your choice of remedy by taking into account such subjective experiences as fear, anger, reactions to people and noise, feeling worse or better in warm or cold surroundings, etc., look them up, together with any other symptoms, in one of the many available books on homoeopathic self-help (SEE *Further Reading*).

This approach is also helpful when you feel under the weather in a non-specific sort of way and are reluctant to 'bother' your GP. You will find remedies for such problems as a bitter taste in the mouth, a suffocating sensation, an aversion to people, being adversely affected by noise, light, smells, etc., dull hair and feeling exhausted after a night's sleep. Choose the remedy that crops up most often in your efforts to link remedies with symptoms. But please bear in mind that vague symptoms *can* be warning signs of an underlying complaint requiring professional diagnosis and treatment. Be sure to consult a medically qualified doctor or homoeopath for any problems that linger despite home remedies.

Homoeopathic Remedies

There are now more than 3,000 homoeopathic remedies and those available for self-treatment are generally in centesimal potencies as already described, for example Arnica 6c. But it is also possible to obtain some of them as mother tinctures and as decimal potencies (dilutions by a factor of 10). The 6c potencies tend to work best for acute (self-limiting) complaints and the 30c potencies for chronic conditions and emergencies. Most remedies are sold as small lactose (milk sugar) pills impregnated with the potentized solution, which you dissolve on your tongue without handling them. You can also buy the liquid to drop directly onto your tongue, to avoid taking lactose, and purchase other remedies as creams and ointments to apply locally.

Here is a selection of homoeopathic remedies in common use:

o *Apis mellifica* – from the bodies or stings of bees, it is useful for painful, swollen insect bites and stings, for allergic reactions and for chickenpox and similar rashes.

o *Arnica* – from leopard's bane; *the* remedy for accidents and emergencies, especially for stalwart people who rarely complain and who pick themselves up after a fall (literally and metaphorically). Good after tumbles, sprains, dental treatment and surgery.

o *Belladonna* – from deadly nightshade. A remedy for violent pains that arise and subside quickly. Suitable for migraines and for the sudden feverish symptoms of children's illnesses. Typical patients tend to be very hot and thirsty.

o *Gelsemium* – from yellow jasmine. Useful for over-excitement and nerviness, for example after an accident or before an examination or other ordeal. The person may feel trembly or leaden and dull, with a dull headache.

o *Hamamelis* – derived from witch hazel bark and, like the herb which has noted astringent properties, it relieves bleeding and bruising from injuries, including nosebleeds. It is also useful for haemorrhoids (piles) and varicose veins, especially those that occur during pregnancy. The homoeopathic remedy is also used to treat conjunctivitis.

o *Hepar sulph* – a sulphur compound, useful for heavy colds with a sore throat, aching or 'blocked' ears and swollen glands. The person may have sharp pain and sour perspiration and be over-sensitive and irritable. Also for right-sided headaches aggravated by the cold and draughts.

5

Acupressure

ACUPRESSURE IS AN Eastern school of therapy which uses thumb or finger pressure at key points on the skin's surface to stimulate the body's inherent self-healing powers. According to *Nei Ching* or *The Yellow Emperor's Classic of Internal Medicine*, it originated, as did acupuncture, more than 5,000 years ago in China, when it was discovered that pressing certain points on the body relieved pain both in that area and in other areas too.

According to legend, soldiers recuperating after a battle found that disorders that had bothered them for years frequently cleared up along with their wounds. Naturally this puzzled the physician-sages, who could not account for the phenomenon. However, nearly all war injuries at the time were inflicted by stones or arrows, piercing or applying great pressure. Eventually, the physicians were prompted to try experimental pressing and piercing healing techniques on their patients, many of whom were relieved or cured of their disorders.

Since the spread of Chinese Traditional Medicine during the twentieth century, we've become increasingly aware that Eastern diagnostic and treatment methods demand an intuition foreign to us in the West. Our technologically sophisticated age sometimes looks askance at the subtleties of pulse and tongue diagnosis, for example, and at therapies applying digital pressure to certain body parts in order to relieve symptoms elsewhere. The fact is that the early beginnings of acupressure (and acupuncture) were nurtured by physicians with an extraordinary empathy with the body and its works. Just as skilled doctors and therapists nowadays can 'go straight to the root' of pain we ourselves can barely pinpoint, so the earliest acupressure practitioners could detect tiny discrepancies in the bodies of sick people and, experimentally or intuitively, identify the trigger points likeliest to help.

Acupressure relieves and cures many medical conditions and also helps to prevent the development of disease through its positive effects upon the immune system. It is a useful adjunct to orthodox or complementary therapies and, as it is based on holistic principles, it attaches great importance to nutrition, exercise, moderate habits, relaxation and other aspects of a balanced lifestyle.

Holistic Acupressure

According to Traditional Chinese medical theory, acupressure works by redressing imbalances in the body's subtle energy or Vital Force, which they regard as the cause of all physical and mental ill health. This energy, known as Ch'i, runs along invisible channels, or meridians (French for 'channel'; acupuncture was first introduced from the East into France) which flow over the body's surface and into its substance to the organs.

When the course of Ch'i runs smoothly and freely, a person remains healthy, with high levels of energy and vitality. When the flow is impeded, however (in Chinese philosophy, when the two great opposing forces of Yin and Yang become unbalanced), then a person's inner rhythms of biological, mental and spiritual function become upset. Ch'i ceases to flow uninhibitedly along the meridians and the effects become noticeable in the appearance of symptoms.

Yin and Yang are essential elements in all Eastern medical theory. They are polar opposites, present in all things, and evidence of them can be perceived everywhere by the practised eye. Familiar, everyday examples of their manifestation include male and female, good and evil, Heaven and Hell, heat and cold, activity and passivity, dryness and wetness.

Within the healthy person, or any living organism, Yin and Yang are in a state of dynamic equilibrium. Far from being 'set' or 'static' (the antithesis of the Eastern concept of health), the influence of each varies slightly from moment to moment in a fluctuating but balanced state like a person walking along a tightrope. One false step and the tightrope walker topples to one or other side, losing their balance and falling (hopefully!) into the safety net. This damaged equilibrium and the resultant descent is analogous to the acupressurist's view of disease. The art and objective of the practitioner is to identify and correct the problem, so restoring health and vitality.

Acupressure is highly suitable for self-treatment; but many therapists also practise it and a brief description of their approach will help to illustrate its underlying concepts.

In assessing a patient and planning treatment, the therapist considers the individual's current and past health problems, lifestyle, diet and stress factors, and the Yin and Yang aspects of the vital organs, together with the elements in nature with which they are associated. Physical examination includes the condition of the nails, the skin colour, the quality of the voice, the state of the tongue, eyes, breathing, posture and emotions, and the patient's body odour.

Diagnosis is based on five colours and five smells. Pulse examination is a very important and highly developed art in Chinese Traditional Medicine. Six can be detected in each wrist, one for each of the 12 main meridians and each linked to a vital organ. Each of the 12 pulses in turn has 24 different qualities. Systematic examination of the pulses provides information about the whereabouts of blocked meridians and whether Yin or Yang is present in excess.

There are 59 meridians in all, dotted throughout their lengths with more than 1,000 acupressure or 'potent' points – tiny invisible dot-like skin areas where Ch'i blockages tend to occur. It is at these points that pressure stimuli have maximum effect.

Proof of the points

'Potent points' have been identified by electrical rather than by anatomical properties; for instance, they have a high voltage compared with surrounding skin and they are highly sensitive to bioelectrical changes, which they readily transmit. With the help of specially adapted apparatus, more than 4,000 of these loci have been traced, of which the traditional 1,000 have been confirmed as a definitive subset. Meridians, too, have been identified by their distinctive electrical properties.

Pain reduction and healing

Research has shown that therapeutic pressure applied to the points releases endorphins, the body's natural pain-relieving chemicals. This is described as 'closing the gates', because it sets up barriers to the habitual passage of pain from an area or organ up the spinal cord to the brain's sensory area. When the pain is relieved, muscles relax, blood, oxygen and nutrients flow more easily and waste metabolites are removed from the affected area, all of which are fundamental to the healing process.

Harmonizing action

The balancing effects which Traditional Chinese Medicine attributes to acupressure can also be explained in Western terms.

Tension accumulates around the potent points and by abolishing pain and spasm, acupressure counteracts the adverse effects of stress. Sustained reduction in tension in one or several body areas boosts the immune defence system, helping it to subdue incipient diseases and prevent others.

Endorphins are also the substances responsible for a 'runner's high', the euphoria generated by aerobic exercise. This may help to explain the improved relaxation, energy and well-being which acupressure users experience.

Relieving ailments

In common with acupuncture, acupressure is unlikely to help conditions where irreversible tissue damage has occurred, such as age-related deafness, glaucoma (an eye complaint), hair loss involving the death of hair follicles, fungal nail infections, and myocardial (heart muscle) damage after a coronary thrombosis (heart attack). But where the condition is amenable to improvement, acupressure can be very effective.

Pain of all types is amenable, including period pain, trigeminal neuralgia, neuralgia (nerve pain) following shingles, stiff, swollen joints and muscles, migraines and other headaches. High blood pressure, hiatus hernia symptoms, stress-related indigestion, irritable bowel, minor bouts of nausea, vomiting and motion sickness, colic and diarrhoea all respond. At a psychological level, pre-examination nerves, panic attacks, anxiety-generated asthma attacks, chronic anxiety, nervous cough or similar habits, insomnia, abnormal appetite and depression may also be relieved.

Working on the Points

Treating an acupressure point can relieve pain or tension in the affected area and/or elsewhere in the body, in which case it is known as a 'trigger point'. Messages sent to other body areas and organs, through bioelectrical impulses passing along interconnecting meridian pathways, means that each point has 'trigger' actions and can potentially relieve a range of problems. The Sea of Energy point, for example, two finger-widths below the navel, relieves allergies linked to constipation, bowel gas, fatigue, general weakness and insomnia.

Each point has a location number which acupressure therapists use as part of a standard reference system, but they are unnecessary for the purpose of self-treatment. Instead, Part II of this book provides each point's traditional name, referring to its location or action, and a brief description of its whereabouts. The Three Mile Point, for example, four finger-widths below the kneecap towards the outside of the shinbone, is said to provide the user with an extra three miles of energy! It is used extensively by sportsmen and women and others in need of extra stamina.

You can maximize the benefits of acupressure by breathing deeply, repeating the name of a point as you apply pressure and picturing the poetic image that comes to into your mind.

Points near a bone usually lie in a small hollow, while those located below major muscle groups can be found in a tendon or ligament, a band of muscle or a knot of tension. Pressure is applied within the indentation or on the muscle part closest to the described point, where most of the pain and tension can be detected, in the following ways:

Firm pressure – using thumbs, fingers, palms or sides of hands or knuckles to apply steady pressure. To relax tension or relieve pain, gradually build the pressure up and hold it without moving for several minutes. This is of benefit to the nervous system and encourages the healing process. Conversely, applying pressure for 4–5 seconds at a time energizes and stimulates the area.

Slow-motion kneading – a kneading action like that used in making bread, this utilizes the thumbs, fingers and heels of the hands to press upon large muscle groups. Lean into the muscle as you apply pressure, to loosen it up. This helps muscular stiffness, neck and shoulder tension, calf muscle cramp and constipation.

Quick tapping – to tone and energize muscles and nerves. Use fingertips on vulnerable areas like the face and a loose fist on areas such as the back or buttocks.

Brisk rubbing – improves the circulation of blood and lymph to the skin and other areas; also relieves swelling, the effects of cold and some forms of numbness.

Hints and tips

- You can practise acupressure almost anywhere; but the ideal is a quiet, peaceful environment. Sit, lie or kneel in the position allowing you maximum unstrained access to the point(s) to be worked on.

- Keep your nails short and wear loose comfortable clothing.

- Wait at least an hour after eating before starting self-treatment. However, you can work safely whenever you need to on hiccups, wind, indigestion or similar minor ailments.

- Unless instructed otherwise, use your middle finger on the points or a small firm ball or similar object if your fingers are painful or weak.

- Apply sustained pressure directly on the point at a 90 degree angle to the skin – if you are dragging the skin, then your approach angle is wrong.

- Initially, work for around three minutes on the points.

- Your goal is the 'it hurts but it's nice' sensation – stop if it becomes too painful. Press as hard as you like on large muscle groups like the buttocks, but treat vulnerable structures such as the throat, temples, the sides of the neck, the genitals and the breasts with great sensitivity.

- Never shove, jab or jar! Gradually increase the pressure slowly and rhythmically, visualizing the various tissue layers through which the stimulus is being transmitted. This helps to keep your mind on the job!

- Always apply and release pressure *gradually* to avoid shocking the tissues and to encourage healing.

- Repeated three-minute pressure sessions may eventually reveal a pulse at the point – a sign that the circulation has improved. If the pulse appears irregular in rate or thrust, you can steady it by pressing for a little longer and noting the effects.

- The pain focus may also move with repeated treatments. Follow and treat it until it diminishes or a clear steady pulse can be detected.

- Stroke the skin gently after treating an area to ease it back to normal.

- Use self-treatment acupressure daily or three to four times weekly to keep fit or relieve an ailment. Maintain the treatment for a couple of weeks after recovering to reduce the risks of recurrence.

- Limit treatment sessions to an hour at the outside. You will be able to sustain pressure on points for longer as you progress, but you should never exceed 10 minutes per point or work on one bodily area for more than 15 minutes.

- If you overdo it, i.e. if the effects are too powerful for your current state of health or for the area or organ concerned, you could experience nausea, headaches or other minor symptoms.

- Avoid direct pressure to traumatized areas such as burns, ulcers, wounds, recent injuries and scars, and operation sites that have not yet healed. Gentle pressure adjacent to the area will encourage healing.

- You may feel shivery after a treatment, in which case wrap up warmly and sip a cup of herbal tea if liked. You should avoid iced drinks and alcohol for several hours after acupressure.

For a list of acupressure points and their location, see the *Appendix*.

6

Yoga

AT ONE LEVEL, Yoga is a movement therapy involving a number of postures, or asanas, that require stretching and bending, carefully co-ordinated with breathing and performed in a studied, calm manner devoid of hurry or strain. In truth, Yoga is a great deal more than this: it is a system of life philosophy that seeks to harmonize body, mind and spirit. There are many schools of Yoga, but the practice as a whole originated in India around 4000 BC and has become increasingly popular in the West since the 1960s.

You may have never thought of Yoga as therapy. Most people learn it from a qualified teacher, and there is no therapist as such. You become your own therapist, obtaining from your regular practice the life qualities of which you are most in need. Yoga strengthens the mind, body and spirit, and its most tangible benefit is improved physical and mental integration, i.e. mind functioning in a way that enhances the physical body rather than sapping its energy, and vice versa. As a result, you experience better health, inner peace, a less extreme, more philosophical attitude to life, an increased capacity to cope with stress, and almost certainly an enhanced awareness of the spiritual world.

Yoga's ultimate goal, from the esoteric standpoint, is the 'fusion of the gross material (annamaya), physical (pranamaya), mental (manomaya), intellectual (vijnanamaya) and spiritual (anandamaya) levels within an individual's being'. More prosaically, this cohesiveness or integration brings about greater resistance to disease, a reduced susceptibility to passing infections, more stamina, more equable emotions, improved memory and concentration, a better relationship with the world, increased self-confidence and self-worth, and, depending on your views, a heightened awareness of spiritual matters.

Holistic Yoga

Yoga can be practised simply as movement therapy, but there is a powerful meditative element to its holistic practice which also encourages healthy eating, fresh air and temperate habits.

Yoga's holistic nature is also apparent in its recognition of the individual self; indeed, self-realization is one of its goals on the spiritual plane. And it offers tangible benefits at physiological, psychological and spiritual levels.

Physiological aspects

Research has shown that Yoga acts upon the brain, nerves and endocrine glands which control the function of tissues and organs throughout the body. It boosts the immune system, helping to prevent diseases and overcoming diseases already present. Interestingly, evidence of its physiological effects comes from the scientifically confirmed achievements of Yoga masters.

Anecdotal evidence over the centuries has confirmed the ability of Yogis to spend hours or days buried in the earth, immersed in icy water or meditating in remote caves. While few of us may wish to do likewise, we now know such feats to be possible through the conscious (Yogic) management of autonomic (i.e. involuntary) bodily functions such as the heartbeat, temperature control, blood pressure and need for oxygen.

These rare accomplishments help to explain how ordinary, 'leisure centre' Yoga can relieve disorders ranging from diabetes, chronic fatigue syndrome, arthritis, hypertension and circulatory problems to digestive complaints, chronic anxiety, migraine and other headaches, varicose veins and asthma. Studies by Yoga institutions in India have shown that asthma attacks can often be avoided, or at least terminated prematurely, in patients practising Yogic postures (asanas) and breathing techniques (pranayama.) Patients suffering from other forms of respiratory disorder, including severe shortness of breath, have also benefited.

High blood pressure often responds satisfactorily to Yoga's combination of exercise, relaxation and improved weight control. Research has shown that Yogic breathing and relaxation combined with biofeedback techniques can reduce both elevated blood pressure and the prescribed doses of antihypertensive drugs.

Yoga has been shown to work in a comparable way to acupressure and acupuncture in its effect on pain, i.e. through the release of endorphins and the gate-controlling mechanism inhibiting the passage of pain signals to the brain. The improved breathing, muscular relaxation and reduced inner tension brought about by Yoga also reduce pain perception, as does the meditative aspect, which greatly reduces anxiety.

Relaxation and Yoga asanas can be particularly helpful for back pain, because of the reduction in tension and improved muscular strength and posture. Combined with deep breathing, they can also ease the stiffness and pain of arthritis, although they should not be practised during an acute inflammatory phase.

Yoga also combats obesity and encourages weight loss. Its overall effect is to improve the circulation of blood and lymph: the former delivers oxygen promptly around the body for the conversion of food calories into energy and the utilization of stored fat, while the latter removes the toxins which encourage the formation of cellulite.

More specifically, several of the asanas, such as the Shoulder Stand and the Fish, stimulate the thyroid gland in the neck which controls the body's metabolism. An underactive thyroid produces a low metabolic rate (rate of burning food fuel) and the accumulation of fat. The reduction in stress and inner turmoil gained from regular Yoga also aids weight loss by combating such stress-fuelled habits as heavy drinking and comfort eating.

Psychological aspects

Depending upon your state of health, your mood, stress levels and/or cognitive function could benefit as much as your physical health from practising Yoga.

○ *Clinical depression*, for example, can make it hard to follow new pursuits, but the combination of daily asanas and breathing exercises raises endorphin levels and increases vitality. Yoga classes also bring you into contact with like-minded people (however unsociable you may feel), while the effort involved in attending them puts you back in control and can bring a precious sense of achievement.

○ *Anxiety and stress*: You can learn from Yoga how to relax at will and cope better with traffic jams, minor accidents, lost car keys and bickering partners/children/colleagues. Premenstrual syndrome (PMS), especially the irritability and the mood swings, menopausal symptoms, phobias, ADHD (attention deficit hyperactivity disorder), obsessive-compulsive disorder and other anxiety-linked problems also benefit from the stress-reduction effects of Yoga.

o *Cognitive improvement* can be seen in better short-term memory and concentration and more mental stamina for studying, revising, learning lines, homework, etc. and for the mental arithmetic, problem-solving and routine paperwork nearly all of us have to perform every day of our lives. Research into brain function and Yoga, including EEGs (electrical tracings of the brain waves), suggest that this enhanced cognition may be connected with the Yoga breathing technique which utilizes one nostril at a time. It seems that this technique stimulates the opposite side of the brain and it is believed that breathing through alternate nostrils facilitates communication between the left and right cerebral hemispheres, improving intellectual powers.

Spiritual aspects

Yoga's spiritual benefits are subjective, therefore more readily experienced than described. Inner peace, feeling at one with yourself and with others, and the enhanced vitality and well-being that follow integration of mind and body are all aspects of this.

At an esoteric level, various schools of Yoga (for example Hatha Yoga, Kundalini Yoga) include practices concentrating on the seven psychic centres or chakras within the body to generate a spiritual power known as kundalini energy. Kundalini, meaning 'coiled up' in Sanskrit, is the potential form of prana or life force, pictured as a serpent coiled up within the first chakra at the base of the spine.

The objective is to awaken the kundalini then raise it upwards through successive chakras via three psychic channels running alongside the spinal cord. When the kundalini reaches the seventh chakra in the crown of the head, self-realization is attained, inducing bliss (Samadhi) and wisdom or illumination (Jnana).

> **CAUTION:** Potent, potentially dangerous forces can be released in raising the kundalini and it should only be attempted when the student of Yoga is ready and under expert guidance.

Yoga Asanas

Here is a list of Yoga asanas and the ailments they can relieve.

> **CAUTION:** Before undertaking any of these asanas, check your fitness and suitability.

- Bow
- Cobra
- Complete Breath
- Corpse
- Eye and Neck Exercises
- Fish
- Grip
- Knee in Chest
- Knee to Chest
- Kneeling Pose
- Lion
- Locust
- Mountain

o Plough

o Posterior Stretch

o Shoulder Roll

o Shoulder Stand

o Sun Salutation

o Twist

o Uddiyana

o *Asthma* – Complete Breath, Corpse, Fish, Mountain, Shoulder Stand

o *Backache* – Corpse, Knee to Chest, Locust, Plough

o *Constipation* – Corpse, Fish, Knee to Chest (invigorates bowel, spleen and liver), Plough, Posterior Stretch, Twist (loosens and flexes spine), Uddiyana, Yoga Mudra

o *Depression* – Corpse, Plough, Shoulder Stand, Yoga Mudra

o *Exhaustion and lethargy* – Corpse, Mountain, Posterior Stretch, Shoulder Stand

o *Eyestrain* – Neck and Eye Exercises

o *Flatulence* – Knee to Chest

o *Headache* – Corpse, Neck and Eye Exercises, Shoulder Roll

o *Indigestion* – Cobra, Corpse, Locust, Mountain, Plough, Twist, Uddiyana

o *Insomnia* – Cobra, Corpse, Locust, Mountain, Posterior Stretch

o *Obesity* – Bow, Cobra, Locust, Plough, Posterior Stretch, Shoulder Stand, Sun Salutation

○ *Period problems* – Cobra, Fish, Plough, Posterior Stretch, Shoulder Stand

○ *Piles* – Fish, Plough, Shoulder Stand

○ *Prostate gland problems* – Kneeling Pose

○ *Rheumatism* – Knee in Chest, Mountain, Shoulder Stand, Twist

○ *Sciatica* – Grip, Knee in Chest, Kneeling Pose, Shoulder Stand, Twist

○ *Sexual problems* – Complete Breath, Plough, Shoulder Stand, Twist, Uddiyana

○ *Sinusitis* – Corpse, Shoulder Stand

○ *Skin disorders* – Sun Salutation

○ *Sore throat* – Lion

○ *Varicose veins* – Shoulder Stand

○ *Wrinkles* – Shoulder Stand, Yoga Mudra

7

Relaxation and Autohypnosis

W E'VE ALL EXPERIENCED tension headaches or a stiff neck and shoulders when under pressure, but the effects of stress can be insidious. We succumb to colds and flu more readily, cuts and scratches take longer to heal, our low mood dips into depression and we all know of someone contracting shingles, for example, or cancer, following a bad fall, bereavement, car accident or some other trauma. Sadly, we are often so conditioned to stress that we fail to make the connection, but its adverse effects *can* be countered by regular relaxation.

Deep Muscular Relaxation

This exercise reminds you what muscular tension feels like, before creating its opposite – deep muscular relaxation. It consists of contracting then letting go of muscle groups throughout the body, starting with the feet and legs and working upwards to the neck, head, scalp, face and tongue. Feeling tense all over can become habitual and focusing on a 'squeeze–relax' routine pinpoints the muscles most in need of attention. It also stills whirling, anxious thoughts and helps to calm the mind.

Wear loose comfortable clothing – a tracksuit is ideal. Sit in a comfortable chair or lie on a soft rug on the floor. Choose a time when you will be left alone for 20–30 minutes at least and turn off the radio, TV or any other source of noise. When you are more practised, you may like to play gentle music as a relaxation aid.

The routine in the same for each muscle group:

- Tense and hold for 15–20 seconds and note how this feels.

- Say 'Relax' to yourself and let the tension go.

- Focus on the difference in feeling between the two.

- Enjoy the sensation for 20–30 seconds, repeat if necessary and move on to the next group.

Focus on these groups in turn:

Toes/feet: Work on each side in turn. Curl your toes – not hard enough to give you cramp, but hard enough to feel the pull. Then uncurl, relax and move on.

Lower legs: Bend your toes and feet downwards and squeeze, tightening the calf muscles. Next, bend your toes and feet upwards towards your face, tightening the muscles at the front and sides. Relax.

Thighs: Straighten and stiffen your legs, bringing your foot slightly upwards to tense the muscles at the front, then bend slightly at the knee to flex the muscles on the back of the thigh. Relax.

Stomach: Pull in your stomach, then push it out.

Buttocks: Squeeze and relax.

Back: Arch and relax.

Chest: Take deep breath and hold it, let it go and relax.

Arms/hands: Do each in turn. Relax.

Hands and forearms: Make a tight fist, bend downwards the elbow. Relax.

Biceps (front of upper arm): 'Make a muscle.' Relax.

Triceps (back of upper arms): Stretch your arms out straight. Tense the backs of your upper arms. Relax.

Shoulders: Shrug and roll your shoulders backwards and forwards. Let them sag and relax.

Neck: Slowly and gently, roll your head right round in circle, up over your right shoulder, then downwards, up over your left shoulder and upwards to the ceiling or the floor above your head. Relax.

Jaws: Clench and let go. Relax.

Forehead: Frown hard, then raise your eyebrows. Relax.

Lips: Press them together. Relax.

Tongue: Stick it out then put it in and press it against the roof of your mouth. Relax.

You are now ready for:

Total body relaxation

- Check each muscle group in turn and repeat the tensing/letting go routine for any group as required.

- Tell yourself that you feel warm, comfortable and relaxed all over.

- Imagine that you are floating gently down a perfumed stream strewn with rose petals.

- Count down slowly from 10 to 1, enjoying the dappled sunlight, the shade, the birds and the flowers. You are feeling more and more deeply relaxed as you approach a small secret pool where you come gently to rest, perfectly relaxed and at peace.

- Enjoy…

- When you wish to come out of it, say to yourself: 'To wake up, I am going to count from 1 to 10. By the time I reach 10, I shall be wide awake and refreshed. 1 … 2 … 3 … 4 … 5 … I am waking up … 6 … 7 … 8 … I am stretching and opening my eyes … 9 … 10 … I am fully awake and feel wonderful.'

Another Relaxation Method

Here is an alternative relaxation method I devised myself, which is equally simple to use. It works slightly more quickly, but its purpose (second to pleasurable relaxation) is the proof it affords of the mind's control of the body. In this instance, the sensations result from the interplay between the inhibiting conscious mind and the suggestibility of the subconscious.

○ Lie or sit comfortably as before. Once you are calm and still, concentrate on one of your feet – let's say the right. Try to contract its muscles – squeezing toes, bending the foot downwards, etc. – *but, at the same time, prevent any movement from actually taking place.* I say to myself: 'I am squeezing my right foot, but I can't. I am squeezing as hard as I can – but nothing is happening.' You will feel a sort of warm vibration passing through the area on which you are concentrating, as though all the tiny fibres in the targeted muscles are contracting randomly on their own instead of concertedly producing movement, leaving the muscle immobile.

o Now repeat with your left foot, right calf, left calf, right then left thigh, buttocks then stomach muscles and so on, working up your body as before and ending with your tongue. The higher up your body you move, the fainter the trembly, vibratory sensation will become. This doesn't matter – having achieved the sensation in your feet and lower legs, and possibly your thighs, each part in turn will become relaxed.

o It takes me about 6–7 minutes to relax in this way and when I have done so, I repeat calming words or a phrase, drawing them out like this: 'Relaaaaax... Peeeaaaaace, be stiiiiill... Total caaaaalm...' Use these or choose whatever works best for you.

Relax in Moments

Regular relaxation makes it easier to deal with negative stress in general, but what do we do when we're suddenly faced with a stressful situation? Stressful situations can arise without warning – at work, at home, in a shop or the bank, or, worst of all, when we're driving or battling to retain our sanity in the face of automated telephone systems. For the hot-blooded among us, a second or two of intense stress can send our blood pressure soaring, while angry words or tears escape and steam billows out of our ears. Apart from the distress and embarrassment this causes, white-hot rage can be a prelude to a heart attack or stroke. Here's how to remain cool in the face of intolerable stress:

o First, take two or three very slow, very deep breaths. This will slow your heart rate and counteract some of that bounding adrenaline.

○ *Walk away* if it's physically possible, and it nearly always is, except in a traffic jam.

○ Sit down – a loo, a large cupboard, the back garden or a shed are all fine, just sit down *somewhere* as comfortably as you can, continuing to breathe slowly and deeply.

○ Now make use of a small part of your body relaxation routine. Make a tight fist with one or other hand, squeeze hard for a few seconds and direct all your rage, pain or grief into that hand, wrist and forearm. Then, gently, relax.

○ Accompany your actions with the words 'Teeeeense … relaaaaax' in the gentle drawn-out way you have used before.

○ Now 'make a muscle' with your biceps and again, still breathing slowly and deeply, say the words 'Teeeeense … relaaaaax.' Feel the tightness where all your emotion has gathered in the front of your upper arm, followed by the loose limp sensation of relaxation as the emotion drains away.

○ Then repeat, straightening your arm at the elbow, squeezing all the muscles as hard as possible and saying as before: 'Teeeeense … relaaaaax.' Really feel that rage or grief leaving your body as the muscle fibres become limp.

You can prepare this emergency measure by rehearsing it straight after a normal relaxation session. Picture something that normally stresses you getting squeezed into the tightness of your fist, your biceps, your whole arm muscles, and follow each tense squeeze with completely loose, limp, floppy relaxation. The passing of the tension out of each muscle group symbolizes – *and is* – the draining away of your immediate source of stress.

When you really *cannot* walk away, you can make do quite nicely with a clenched fist – as tight as you can, and fairly prolonged – driving all your negative emotion down into the iron-hard muscles ... and then releasing it, letting it all trickle away as you relax. Repeat the words to go with the action under your breath or just say them in your mind.

Autohypnosis

A further technique utilizes 'arm levitation', sometimes used by hypnotherapists to demonstrate the power of hypnosis by making a client's arm rise up without conscious effort. It is also a test of a client's susceptibility to hypnotic suggestion. Most people find it a useful relaxation aid, although some experts claim that it can trigger panic attacks in unusually sensitive people. If you suffer from convulsions or anxiety-related complaints such as panic attacks, hysterical outbursts or unpleasant physical symptoms such as trembling and heavy sweating when under pressure, consult your doctor or a qualified hypnotherapist before trying this or any other autohypnosis technique.

o Lie comfortably with your legs stretched out and ankles slightly apart and your arms and hands stretched out and lying quietly on either side of your body. Make yourself as relaxed and comfortable as possible – you can go through my own relaxation method first if you like – then concentrate on one of your hands. Clench and relax the hand a few times, concentrating upon achieving complete relaxation in its every part.

o Then, when your hand is as limp and floppy as you can make it, say, 'My [left/right] hand is starting to rise. Very, very slowly, without any effort from me, my [left/right] hand is slowly and surely starting to lift up. A helium balloon is attached to my wrist and is slowly but surely carrying my hand upwards without my conscious effort. Slowly but surely, slowly but surely, my hand is rising from the [floor, bed, sofa, whatever].

> It's as light as a feather, as light as gossamer, up it goes upwards, upwards, upwards…'

You are instructing your subconscious mind to carry out an action which you have prohibited your conscious mind from performing. You will probably notice a warm vibratory feeling in your hand muscles similar to the one described in the last exercise. And if you increase the intensity of your suggestions, repeating them over and over, saying them more and more emphatically as the thumb and fingers start to twitch and then move, you will find that your hand – possibly your entire arm – will slowly rise upwards until it is anything from a fraction of a centimetre above the surface on which it has been resting to extended fully above your head, suspended in the air without any conscious effort on your part.

○ With your hand and arm aloft, you can then imagine that you are floating down a stream or on a cloud down a mountainside and can prolong the relaxation for 10–15 minutes. For most of us, however, the unique experience of arm levitation is sufficient achievement at any one time and by the time you have elevated your arm or hand as far as you can, you will have benefited from healing relaxation anyway.

Whichever relaxation method you choose, its regular practice will boost your physical and emotional well-being and work with a mainly wholefood diet and exercise to improve your resistance to many ailments.

In Part II, we look at common ailments affecting each bodily system and at using home remedies to relieve or cure them.

Common Ailments and their Treatment

8

Digestive Ailments

- Abdominal pain • Anal itching • Bleeding gums and bad breath • Colitis • Constipation • Diarrhoea • Difficulty in swallowing • Diverticulitis • Gall bladder inflammation • Gullet spasm • Heartburn/indigestion • Inguinal hernia • Intestinal thrush • Irritable bowel syndrome • Loss of appetite • Mouth ulcers • Piles • Sore mouth or tongue • Stomach upset • Threadworms • Toothache and sensitive teeth • Wind

▪ Abdominal Pain

Abdominal pain may be due to a *stomach upset* or *heartburn/indigestion* or other common causes. Colic produces spasms of pain which reach a pitch, subside and recur. Food poisoning and dysentery (SEE *Diarrhoea*), *irritable bowel syndrome* (*IBS*), *diverticulitis* and *colitis* can all cause colic.

Stomach pain also features in *gall bladder inflammation*, appendicitis, *tonsillitis* (in children under 12 years), menstruation (SEE *Painful Periods*), a kidney or bladder infection and kidney stone. Accompanying symptoms can include nausea, vomiting and *diarrhoea*, aching muscles, *headache*, fever and *loss of appetite*.

WHAT YOU CAN DO

- Encourage normal digestion by eating healthily (SEE *Nutritional Medicine*) and sitting down to meals. Chew your food thoroughly!

- Your appendix can become inflamed when fruit pips get wedged inside it. Avoid swallowing these to minimize the risk.

- Children with *tonsillitis* and tummyache may also have an inflamed appendix. As a rule of thumb, appendicitis pain starts in the centre around your navel, later moving to the lower right quarter of your abdomen just inside your hip bone. It is rare, though not unknown, for *diarrhoea* to co-exist with appendicitis. If abdominal pain is appendicitis, the chances are that you will not have opened your bowels on the day that the symptoms appear.

- Avoid fatty foods to calm an irritable gall bladder. This causes pain in the upper right quarter of your abdomen, spreading through to your back near the tip of your right shoulder blade.

- Drink eight glasses of water daily in addition to other drinks. Dehydration encourages stones to form in the kidneys and gall bladder.

- Sip fennel tea made from the fresh or dried herb to soothe painful spasms of the stomach or bowel.

- Try peppermint oil capsules (SEE *Herbal Medicine*) or an *aromatherapy* massage. After a bath or shower, pat yourself dry and use oil to massage your whole abdomen, working clockwise with the flat of your hand using smooth, gentle strokes.

- Try *acupressure*:

  o For bowel cramp, work on the Grandfather, Grandson potent point.

  o For *indigestion*, use Inner Gate.

Drug remedies

(SEE *also Diarrhoea, Gullet Spasm, Heartburn/Indigestion, Stomach Upset.*)

o *Colic:* Peppermint oil capsules, and the anti-spasmodic drug mebeverine hydrochloride, available as capsules, tablets and liquid.

o Powerful painkillers such as pethidine or morphine may be prescribed for intensely painful kidney or gall bladder spasm unrelieved by anti-spasmodics.

o *Dysentery:* The antibiotic metronidazole may be prescribed for amoebic dysentery. Other antibiotics (such as cefradine) are used to treat bacterial dysentery.

SEE YOUR DOCTOR IF...

- Your pain is severe/fails to respond to home treatment.
- You risk becoming dehydrated.
- Vomiting, *diarrhoea*, fever, etc. are distressing or prolonged.
- Home treatments fail to give relief.

▪ Anal Itching

An itchy anus can be due to poor hygiene – perspiration and tiny smears of faeces collecting around the back passage. *Heavy perspiration* is often due to woollen or nylon tights or pants overheating the nether region. Detergents, lavatory paper, perfumed talc or intimate deodorants can also trigger a pricking, tingling allergy rash.

Bowel mucus (SEE *Colitis*) or a *vaginal discharge* in contact with the back passage can cause severe irritation, and an anal fissure – an open split in the anus following powerful straining – causes both itching and soreness.

Diabetes, *intestinal thrush*, lactose intolerance, *threadworms* and some forms of *anxiety* and nervous tension can also produce a need for frequent scratching.

WHAT YOU CAN DO

- Wash your anal area with unscented soap and water morning and night and after opening your bowels. Apply a little antiseptic cream after drying.

- Avoid tights, tight trousers and thongs which can rub and irritate. Wear stockings and cool cotton pants which let the skin breathe.

- Use a non-biological detergent and rinse handwashed garments thoroughly.

- Use plain, soft, white lavatory paper with or without aloe vera, vitamins or other additives.

- Check the symptoms of *intestinal thrush*. Identification and treatment relieves anal itching for many sufferers.

- *Threadworms* (also known as pinworms) typically cause an itchy bottom.

- If emotional tension aggravates your symptoms, try *Yoga*, meditation and/or *relaxation*.

- When plagued by anal itch, run a few inches of cool water into your bathtub, stir in a handful of salt or 3–4 drops of echinacea or tea tree oil and sit with your bottom immersed for 15–20 minutes. Pat yourself dry carefully afterwards and apply one of the following:

  ○ Healing calendula cream (derived from marigolds) has a soothing, anti-inflammatory effect. Alternatively, use a homoeopathic/herbal cream combining extracts of calendula and hypericum (St John's wort), brand name Hypercal, to heal angry skin and itching.

  ○ Add 2–3 drops of essential oil of geranium to your bathwater or 1 drop each of geranium and cypress to a little cold cream and apply as above.

- Homoeopathic remedies to take 4 times daily for up to 14 days:

  ○ For itchiness that also involves the scrotum (testicles) or vulva and gets worse in company: Ambra 6c

  ○ For violent itching and a crawling sensation around the anus, aggravated by warmth: Ignatia 5c

  ○ For itching and smarting which is worse at night, when there is alternating *constipation* and *diarrhoea*, especially if the person is elderly and there is mucous discharge from anus, aggravated by heat, acid foods, water and wine: Antimonium 6c

Drug remedies

○ Antiseptic cream applied to the anus after washing and drying.

○ Anti-inflammatory creams (designed for the anal area) and creams and ointments used to relieve *piles*.

○ Local anaesthetic/astringent creams used to relieve *piles* and anal fissure.

SEE YOUR DOCTOR IF...

- Your home relief methods are not effective.
- You have anal itching and suffer from a *vaginal discharge*, diabetes or lactose intolerance, or suspect you may have *intestinal thrush* or an anal fissure.
- You need professional help for nervous tension – counselling, psychotherapy or hypnotherapy can all offer effective relief.

■ Bleeding Gums and Bad Breath

If blood appears when you brush or floss your teeth or bite a crispy apple, gum disease is surely responsible. It starts when 'normal' mouth bacteria form a sticky deposit on the teeth's surface, react with food sugars and attack the teeth's enamel. Chalky tartar forms around the teeth's base, triggering gum inflammation (gingivitis). Besides bleeding, painful gums, you may have *sensitive teeth*, a bad taste in your mouth and smelly breath.

The next stage is periodontitis, in which the bacteria penetrate more deeply into the gums. Here, they destroy the connective tissue anchoring the teeth and erode the underlying bone. You could experience any or all of the above symptoms with periodontitis, plus oozing pus, loose teeth and eventually dental loss.

WHAT YOU CAN DO

- Combat gum disease in its earliest stages, or prevent it altogether! It causes more loss of teeth than dental decay and recent research at Cardiff University has linked it to an increased risk of heart attacks and *strokes*. Bacteria released into the bloodstream from infected gum crevices during brushing and flossing encourage the fatty clogging of arteries to vital organs.

- Test yourself for bad breath – lick the inside of your wrist, wait 30 seconds for it to dry and then sniff…

- Chew a handful of fresh parsley – the chlorophyll combats offensive breath.

- Brush and floss your teeth after meals to remove plaque and sweeten breath. Replace your brush every 3–4 months for the best results.

- Use toothpastes and mouthwashes containing fluoride to strengthen teeth against decay.

- Use a mouthwash twice daily. Recently introduced 24-hour oral care products called RetarDEX eliminate the volatile sulphur compounds (VSCs) responsible for embarrassing whiffs.

- Use disclosure reagents to reveal tartar build-up.

- Have a dental check-up and visit your dental hygienist every 6–12 months.

- Stop smoking – it actively encourages gum disease!

- Chew sugar-free gum to keep the saliva flowing and combat plaque formation.

- Avoid dehydration and a dry mouth (which enhances bacterial activity) by drinking eight large tumblers of water daily.

- Cut down on sweet foods, fizzy drinks and fruit squashes; brush or rinse afterwards. (Fruit acids can encourage dental decay.)

Drug remedies

○ Take two paracetamol or ibuprofen two to three times daily for aching teeth or gums.

○ Antiseptic mouthwashes (SEE *Sore Mouth or Tongue*) will ease the pain.

○ Your dentist or doctor will prescribe an antibiotic if your gums are infected.

○ Hyaluranon has been shown in five clinical studies significantly to reduce gum bleeding and soreness and promote healing. A natural constituent of gum tissue, which it strengthens and protects while plugging the gap at the tooth–gum juncture, it is attacked by plaque bacteria which break the seal, enabling the inflammation to penetrate more deeply.

○ Hyaluranon is used by dentists in the treatment of gingivitis and is now available for personal use. A natural adhesive, it stays in place and should be applied 3–5 times daily for 3–4 weeks until all symptoms have disappeared. It's safe for use during pregnancy and by children and the elderly, and its natural sweetener makes suitable for diabetics (who are extra prone to gum disease). It is available as Gingivel in the form of a gel for gum application or as a liquid for rinsing from dentists, Boots and major supermarkets.

SEE YOUR DENTIST OR DOCTOR IF...

• You suspect you have gum disease.
• Your bad breath persists despite home measures.

▪ Colitis

If you suffer from colitis (large bowel inflammation), you will be familiar with the *abdominal pain, diarrhoea* and *loss of appetite* it causes. The milder, non-ulcerative variety – sometimes called mucoid – is common, with attacks lasting from a few days to over a week and invariably brought on by stress. The motions can be semi-formed or liquid, contain mucus and/or blood and, distressingly, you may lose control of your bowels when symptoms are acute. Tummy pain, often mild and diffuse at first, eventually settles in the lower abdomen and can be severe.

Ulcerative colitis is a comparatively rare illness in which the colon's lining becomes ulcerated and infected. Pus, blood and mucus appear in the *diarrhoea*, and skilled medical treatment is needed to help prevent weight loss, anaemia, septicaemia and other possible complications. It is an autoimmune complaint but attacks are triggered by *anxiety* and stress.

WHAT YOU CAN DO

- Take stock of your life and pinpoint aggravating stress factors. Aim at eliminating as many as possible.

- Take active measures to cope with unavoidable stress. Consider counselling, psychotherapy or hypnotherapy if appropriate and take up *Yoga, relaxation* and/or *autohypnosis.*

- Here are some beneficial *acupressure* points:

  o Crooked Pond

  o Three Mile Point

- Try *Bach Flower Remedies.* Suitable choices could be Oak, which combats despondency when faced with difficult situations, and Vervain if you are unable to relax.

- Stop smoking.

- Avoid any food or drink that tends to worsen your symptoms. Avoid alcohol, red meat, tea and coffee and cola drinks, and cut down on dairy products until the attack subsides. Stick to wholefoods, limiting your intake of fibre (in fresh fruit and vegetables, wholegrains and their products) until recovery is really under way.

- Try a liquids-only routine for 24–48 hours – 6–8 glasses of mineral water a day plus diluted non-citrus fresh fruit and vegetable juices. Follow with bland, soft, comforting foods such as scrambled eggs, minced turkey breast, steamed white fish and tofu.

- Drink 100–300 ml of freshly squeezed cabbage juice 3 times daily for its healing action on your inflamed bowel lining.

- Take 1 tbsp aloe vera gel or liquid 3 times daily (or follow package directions).

- Eat live yoghurt or take an acidophilus supplement once or twice daily.

- Medical herbalists may prescribe lavender, lime flowers, mallow and marjoram. You can add handfuls of the fresh herbs to bath-water, sip lime-flower tea (which soothes the nerves) or add 2–3 drops of aromatherapy essence of marjoram and/or lavender to your bath.

- Homoeopathic remedies to take every 2 hours up to 10 doses for acute symptoms while you are waiting for other measures to work:

  ○ For bloody stools, when passing stools relieves the pain but the anus feels wide open afterwards: Phosphorus 6c

  ○ For hot offensive stools containing mucus and blood, cutting pains on opening the bowels and no relief afterwards: Mercurius corr. 6c

Drug remedies

○ Anti-spasmodic drugs such as mebeverine, or an anti-diarrhoeal drug such as loperamide or diphenoxylate.

○ Codeine compounds calm colicky spasm and curb *diarrhoea.* Paracetamol + codeine is available from pharmacies or (with a higher codeine content) on prescription.

SEE YOUR DOCTOR IF...

- You develop fever or see pus or large drops of blood in your stools.
- You suspect you have ulcerative colitis.
- Your symptoms are not helped by home treatments.

■ Constipation

Medically, constipation means opening your bowels less often than usual. Many 'regular' people become anxious when their routine is disturbed, but there is nothing dangerous about a few days of bowel sluggishness. Fretting merely compounds the problem.

Besides passing fewer motions, constipation can involve a struggle to pass hard stools. Causes include too little exercise, becoming dehydrated, a change in the balance between friendly and unfriendly bowel bacteria and too little fibre in the diet. If you have *irritable bowel syndrome (IBS)*, you're likely to suffer from constipation and *diarrhoea* in turn, together with flatulence (SEE *Wind*), bloating and tummy pain. Diet, depression and an inherited tendency may all be responsible.

WHAT YOU CAN DO

- Go to the lavatory when the need arises. Postponement allows faeces to build up, becoming dry and hard. A frequently over-loaded gut wall loses elasticity. It then becomes insensitive to the normal stimuli leading to waste expulsion.

- Take regular gentle exercise. Walking, cycling, swimming, dancing and aquarobics all encourage regular bowel habits.

- Try *Yoga*: Recommended asanas include the Corpse, Fish, Knee to Chest, which reinvigorates the liver, spleen and bowel, Plough and Twist, which mobilizes the pelvis.

- Cut down on refined foods and eat more fibre-rich wholefoods. Fresh and dried figs, rhubarb, carrots and butternut squash are natural laxatives. Cook the latter as you would pumpkin or add it to casseroles or soups. Introduce changes gradually, to avoid a *stomach upset*.

- Drink 2 litres (3 pints) of water daily to help keep your stools moist.

- Stock up internally with friendly bacteria – eat plain, live yoghurt daily or take one of the flora-rich yoghurt-type drinks available in healthfood shops and supermarkets.

- Medical herbalists may recommend extra fibre in the form of ispaghula husks, oat or wheat bran, or 15 ml (1tbsp) extra virgin olive oil daily, which acts as a lubricant.

- Delicious liquorice is a popular and effective constipation remedy. Chew some liquorice 'shoelaces' or suck a juice stick, available from delicatessens and healthfood shops.

CAUTION: Avoid liquorice if you take the heart drug digoxin or have high blood pressure.

- Lie down and massage your abdomen with marjoram and/or rosemary essential oils.

Drug remedies

○ Bulk laxatives – made up into drinks, they expand in the bowel and stimulate movement.

○ Lactulose – a sugary solution which works by attracting fluid into the bowel by osmosis. Hard stools absorb water and the increased bulk triggers the bowel wall into action.

○ Senna (from herbal senna pods) irritate the bowel lining, sparking contractions to expel faeces.

SEE YOUR DOCTOR IF...

- You experience a significant change in bowel habit. Constipation or *diarrhoea* or periods of one alternating with the other over weeks or months may mean something is amiss and needs to be investigated.
- Home remedies do not help.

■ Diarrhoea

Diarrhoea demands immediate attention and can be impossible to conceal. It can run a lone course or accompany *abdominal pain* and vomiting due to food poisoning (SEE *Stomach Upset*). Many people develop 'the runs' when anxious or upset. Diarrhoea is also a feature of *irritable bowel syndrome*, food sensitivity, *colitis, diverticulitis*, alcohol abuse and carbohydrate intolerance, and can develop as a side-effect to medication, for example NSAIDs (non-steroidal anti-inflammatory drugs such as ibuprofen).

Diarrhoea symptoms can include numerous dashes to the lavatory, passing liquid or semi-liquid stools, *wind*, griping tummy pain, bloating, a dry mouth and *loss of appetite*. Streaks of blood may appear in your stools during a violent attack. A sore rectum and anus can follow heavy drinking, when the diarrhoeic stools are laden with the irritating breakdown products of alcohol.

WHAT YOU CAN DO

Prevention

- Avoid large quantities of alcohol, rich, fatty or highly spiced dishes, fizzy drinks, sugar and foods to which you are intolerant.

- When abroad, avoid tap water and cooked or raw food sold on open stalls. Wash and peel fruit and choose cooked food when eating out in preference to (possibly unwashed) salads.

- If emotional tension is the cause, seek help from counselling or other forms of psychotherapy, *Yoga* or *relaxation*.

If you do succumb

- Avoid solid foods for 24 hours and sip an isotonic sports drink such as Lucozade Sports. Blueberries and their juice or tea combat large bowel inflammation. (SEE *also the mixture suggested for vomiting in Stomach Upsets.*)

- Watch for signs of dehydration – a dry mouth, a bad taste in the mouth, pallor and loss of skin elasticity.

- *Rest* if you have severe diarrhoea. Nursing a hot water bottle can help to soothe painful spasms. Take codeine or another pharmaceutical to relieve diarrhoea and colic.

- Herbs prescribed to treat diarrhoea and colic include powdered slippery elm and marshmallow.

- Sip cinnamon or lime-flower tea or use aloe vera juice or gel to calm an inflamed colon.

- Massage your abdomen using essential oil of benzoin, black pepper, fennel or ginger to relieve painful spasms.

- Try these homoeopathic remedies at 30-minute intervals for up to 10 doses:

  o For diarrhoea which is worse at night and after cold drinks and oily food: Pulsatilla 6c

  o For severe colic which starts and stops suddenly, when symptoms are worsened by movement and jarring: Belladonna 30c

Drug remedies

o Pharmaceutical fluid and electrolyte replacements guard against dehydration and can sometimes quell an attack without other medicines.

o Loperamide is a useful treatment for occasional diarrhoea.

o Diphenoxylate, also effective, is available on prescription.

SEE YOUR DOCTOR IF...

- Pain is severe.
- You see spots (rather than small specks) of blood in your stools. Blood mixed in with the stools and/or black or dark in colour comes from higher up the digestive tract and the cause needs to be established.
- Fluids 'go right through you' without the attack abating.
- You suffer from recurrent diarrhoea (or other change in bowel habit) for no known reason.
- The symptoms are unrelieved by home treatments.

▪ Difficulty in Swallowing

We've all experienced a 'lump in the throat' when emotional, but true difficulty in swallowing lasts longer. *Tonsillitis* and other throat infections are the most common causes, along with scalds and injury caused by hot foods and drinks, gulping down large tablets with too little water (thereby bruising the throat) and swallowing a hard food or a foreign body (SEE *Sore Throat*).

Vomiting can chemically burn your throat by bringing stomach acid into contact with its lining. Smoke inhalation is a consequence of fires and although damage to the air tubes is generally the greatest concern, the throat can also suffer. When, rarely, a tumour of the gullet or oesophagus is responsible for swallowing difficulties, you will probably first experience difficulty with swallowing liquids and then later with solids. Spasm of the throat muscles can also occur if you are very tense and stressed. *Stroke* patients and others with neurological problems are also prone to dysphagia, the medical name for swallowing difficulty.

WHAT YOU CAN DO

- Make any of the drinks for gargling and/or sipping mentioned under *Sore Throat*. Sage tea is also beneficial.

- Stick to bland soft foods which cannot hurt your throat, such as jelly, ice cream, puréed vegetables and non-citrus fruit, and milk puddings.

- Chew some fresh or crystallized angelica. Avoid at bedtime, as it can act as a stimulant.

- To soothe a throat aggravated by vomiting, gargle with and sip 5 ml (1 level tsp) bicarbonate of soda (cooking soda) mixed into half a tumbler of cold water.

- For throat scalds and other minor injuries, sip and gargle with aloe vera liquid to reduce inflammation and pain.

- Peppermint oil relieves spasm throughout the digestive tract. Make the herbal tea or buy capsules of the oil from a pharmacist to take by mouth. Inhaling peppermint essential oil is also beneficial.

- If tension and stress are the cause, practise *relaxation* or *auto-hypnosis* or take regular exercise for its calming effects.

Drug remedies

o Paracetamol or an anti-inflammatory medication such as nurofen should provide satisfactory pain relief. (Only take the latter if you have been entirely free from stomach or bowel discomfort when you have taken it in the past.)

o Swallow one of the proprietary antacids – your pharmacist will stock a selection.

o Steroid drugs are often prescribed for the injury caused by smoke inhalation.

SEE YOUR DOCTOR IF...

- *Immediately* if there has been significant smoke inhalation.
- Blood appears in your saliva or at the back of your throat.
- The pain is severe and/or you unsure how much damage you have suffered.
- You have something stuck in your throat.
- You have difficulty in swallowing for more than a few days and for no apparent reason.
- Minor symptoms persist despite home remedies.

▪ Diverticulitis

Diverticulosis refers to little blind finger-like projections of the lining membrane of the large bowel which push out through weak spots in the muscular walls. If you have these pouches – diverticula – you may experience occasional cramps and tenderness in the lower left abdomen, relieved by passing stools or *wind*, plus bouts of *diarrhoea, constipation* and occasional blood in the stools.

If the pouches become infected and inflamed, the condition is called diverticulitis and you are likely to have more severe pain, fever and nausea, and run the risk of abscess formation (SEE *Abscesses and Boils*) and peritonitis (inflammation of the abdominal lining) due, in this case, to a ruptured abscess.

Diverticulitis therefore has a number of features in common with *irritable bowel syndrome*, but IBS does not typically produce a fever, and simple tests can distinguish between the two. An endoscopy ('magic eye'), a barium enema or a scan should all reveal diverticula in the lower portion of the colon. Reasons for their formation include an inherited weakness in the bowel wall and prolonged straining to open the bowels (SEE *Constipation*).

WHAT YOU CAN DO

- Avoid becoming constipated – hard dry stool pellets can get stuck in the pouches and cause infection, while straining encourages diverticula formation. Aim for a high roughage diet with plenty of fresh fruit and vegetables, wholegrain products and their flour, and avoid sugary, fatty, low-fibre junk and convenience foods.

- Take regular gentle exercise and drink six to eight glasses of water daily.

- Psyllium husks, 1–2 tsp or the equivalent in capsules, should be taken with water daily while needed.

- Make up some cinnamon massage oil and massage your abdomen after a warm bath.

- Relieve nausea with ginger tea. Place a sachet or a small piece of grated fresh ginger root into a mug of boiling water, allow to cool for 5–10 minutes and strain before sipping. Enhance the flavour by stirring it with a cinnamon stick or adding a pinch of the ground spice – cinnamon is powerfully antiseptic and regulates the gut's muscle tone.

- Here are some valuable *acupressure* points:

  o Joining the Valley (Hoku)

> **CAUTION:** Avoid if pregnant because stimulation can cause premature contractions.

  o Sea of Energy
  o Three Mile Point

Drug remedies

  o Bulk laxatives, for example ispaghula husks or psyllium husks, to avoid or treat constipation. These work by increasing the bulk of the stools, which gets the bowel moving, and this in turn increases the diameter of the colon, thereby reducing the pressure within (high inner bowel pressure encourages diverticula to form).

  o Painful spasms generally respond to an anti-spasmodic drug such as mebeverine.

  o Antibiotics may be prescribed when fever and infection are present.

SEE YOUR DOCTOR IF...

- *Abdominal pain*, nausea, *constipation* or *diarrhoea* cause undue distress.
- Fever and/or an intensely tender abdomen suggest you may be developing complications.
- Home treatments fail to work.

■ Gall Bladder Inflammation

Calcium, cholesterol and other substances present in bile can come out of solution within the gall bladder and form gall stones. While these remain in the cavity of this gland, they cause few symptoms. But if one lodges within the bile duct (the small tube transporting bile to the duodenum or small bowel), the gall bladder swells with trapped bile and becomes inflamed. This, together with undigested fat in the duodenum, gives you the characteristic symptoms of gall bladder inflammation (cholecystitis). These include severe upper right-sided *abdominal pain* extending through to your back (usually the tip of the right shoulder blade) and pronounced tenderness below your right ribs. You probably feel sick, may vomit and may be able to relate your attack to a chocolate binge or rich fatty meal. You're more at risk of developing gall stones if you have taken oral contraceptives, and the risk increases with age and surplus weight.

WHAT YOU CAN DO

- Shed surplus weight, especially if you are female, over forty and have taken or do take the Pill.

- Have your cholesterol level checked – very high levels increase the risks of developing gall stones, as well as heart disease and *stroke*.

- Cut rich fatty foods, fried dishes and refined carbohydrates down to a minimum and fill up on fresh fruit and vegetables plus other sources of healthy fibre.

- Lipotropic compounds help to prevent fat build-up in the liver and encourage liver cells to make lecithin. This helps to prevent cholesterol from forming into gall stones. Common lipotropics include the amino acid methionine, B vitamins inositol and choline and the enzyme betaine. Some nutritionists also recommend supplements of vitamin C and magnesium to discourage gall-stone formation.

- Avoid dehydration – drink six to eight glasses of water every day.

- Homoeopathic remedies to take 4 times a day for up to 14 days while seeking homoeopathic or other personal treatment:

  o Berberis 6c

  o If Berberis does not help, or if the person is nervous, over-sensitive and feeling chilly: China 6c

- Herbal practitioners may recommend treatments with artichoke, barberry (*Berberis vulgaris*), chicory, dandelion, dog's tooth roots, fringe tree and/or poppy petals. A herbal tea infusion of lovage can relieve gall bladder problems by helping to detoxify the body after a food or alcohol binge: drink three to four cups daily.

- You can also inhale the aromatherapy essence Scots pine or add it to your bathwater.

- Chinese research suggests that acupuncture can discharge large gall stones in the motions.

- *Acupressure* experts maintain that excessive physical exertion can damage the gall bladder and liver meridians (energy pathways), giving rise to cramps and spasms. Learn to relax thoroughly and recuperate after vigorous exercise, and massage the Bigger Rushing point to reinvigorate these meridians.

Drug remedies

o Pain relief – paracetamol, NSAIDs (anti-inflammatory drugs like ibuprofen and naproxen), possibly codeine compounds if nausea/vomiting are not a problem.

o Drugs to control nausea and vomiting such as prochlorperazine and metachlopromide.

SEE YOUR DOCTOR IF...

• Your pain/nausea/vomiting are severe.
• Dietary and other relief measures fail to help you.

▪ Gullet Spasm

Spasm of the gullet or oesophagus can cause fear as well as discomfort, because it often mimics *angina*. Doctors also misdiagnose 'diffuse oesophageal spasm' and often an ECG (electrocardiogram) and other tests are needed to distinguish between the two conditions.

If you are a sufferer, you'll be familiar with the intense ache that starts behind the breastbone and spreads up your throat to your lower jaw and teeth. You may also feel light-headed, faint and about to collapse. The vital difference between gullet spasm and *angina* is that the latter is nearly always triggered and aggravated by exercise. Oesophageal spasm is unrelated to exertion, but can be brought on by smoking, stress, strong coffee or tea, spicy foods and long gaps between meals.

WHAT YOU CAN DO

- Avoid strong tea and coffee and spicy foods and eat small snacks as required.

- Do not smoke.

- Counterbalance tension, stress and long periods of concentrated desk work with regular exercise and relaxation.

- When the pain and faintness start, lie down and rest. A short sleep can bring complete relief.

- Avoid dehydration. Sip cool or chilled still or sparkling water frequently.

- If you must have coffee, choose decaffeinated and avoid the strong black stuff. Do not drink coffee on an empty stomach.

- Sip a glass of milk.

- Sip herbal tea – basil, blueberry, chamomile, marjoram, peppermint or sage are good choices. Fennel also relieves gastric spasm. Aloe vera, marshmallow and slippery elm are useful where gastric acid is irritating the symptoms.

- Mint essential oil is helpful – either inhale it or add a few drops to bathwater.

- To relieve stress, try an *aromatherapy* massage. Head, neck and shoulder massage helps banish knots of tension. Try bay laurel, chamomile, clary sage, lavender, marjoram, rose, thyme, verbena and ylang ylang essential oils.

- Try a *Bach Flower Remedy*. Olive can relieve physical and mental exhaustion, Rock Rose reduces panic and Holly counterbalances negative emotions.

Drug remedies

○ Peppermint oil capsules are helpful.

○ *Angina* drugs are sometimes used to treat severe oesophageal spasm. Glyceryl trinitrate comes as a spray, patches, ointment and tablets. Nifedipine (tablets) also relaxes smooth muscle. Both can cause side-effects such as a throbbing headache and flushing, although these tend to disappear with regular use.

SEE YOUR DOCTOR IF...

- Your symptoms persist despite home remedies. (Surgery to divide the fibres of the gullet's muscles may help extremely severe symptoms.)
- You experience sudden and unfamiliar chest pain when oesophageal spasm has already been diagnosed. It is possible to suffer from *angina* or a heart attack as well, and these must be ruled out.

■ Heartburn/Indigestion

Heartburn refers to a fiery pain in your central chest resulting from an inflamed oesophagus (gullet). Like *gullet spasm*, it can spread to your lower throat, but belching and an acidic taste are common features and it does not cause the same faintness and state of near-collapse.

A hiatus hernia is often responsible – this happens when the upper part of the stomach slides up into the chest through its normal opening in the diaphragm, which becomes enlarged or torn. A common trigger is increased abdominal pressure due to obesity, pregnancy and a chronic *cough* and/or *constipation*.

A hiatus hernia allows the acidic stomach contents to swirl around inside the lower end of the gullet, irritating its lining. Regurgitation of partially digested food into the mouth, known as reflux, commonly occurs. Overheated spicy foods aggravate heartburn, as do stress, hurried meals, an unhealthy diet and smoking, all of which increase the stomach's production of acid.

Pain in the centre at the top of your abdomen, just below your breastbone, can be due to a peptic ulcer in the stomach, gullet or duodenum (part of the small bowel).

WHAT YOU CAN DO

- Lose excess weight and seek treatment for a longstanding *cough* or *constipation.*

- Stop smoking.

- Reduce your alcohol intake to the recognized safe limits.

- Eat healthily – small frequent snacks ease pain and inflammation.

- Cut down on acidic foods, fizzy drinks, strong tea and coffee and rich or sugary junk foods.

- Sip low-fat milk and chew liquorice, which has potent ulcer-healing actions.

- Eat some blueberries, or juice a cabbage and sip 300–400 ml (12–16 fl oz) daily on an empty stomach. Take a vitamin/mineral supplement and add two kelp tablets daily – cabbage juice can interfere with the thyroid gland if you have an iodine deficiency.

- Herbs prescribed for *heartburn* and acid reflux include bay leaves, caraway, ginger, marjoram, marshmallow, mint, savory and thyme. Sip aloe vera juice or gel (follow packet instructions) before three main meals and at bedtime, as research studies have shown this combats *heartburn* and ulcer formation. Cook with these herbs or use them fresh for further effect.

- Combat stress with regular exercise, *relaxation* and meditation.

- Do some *Yoga* – helpful asanas include the Corpse, Locust, Mountain, Plough and Twist.

- Try these *acupressure* points:

  o Abdominal Sorrow – This specifically targets ulcer pain, as well as general indigestion, *hiccups*, unbalanced appetite and abdominal cramps.

  o Jumping Circle

  o Sea of Tranquillity

Drug remedies

o Sodium alginate and potassium bicarbonate mixtures relieve reflux and *heartburn*.

o Antacids/anti-flatulents (to combat *wind*) and anti-spasmodic drugs relieve painful spasms.

o Various medications, for example lansoprazole, curtail the stomach's acid production.

o Triple action treatment (two antibiotics, for example metronidazole, amoxicillin and a stomach acid regulator) may be given for 7–14 days if stomach bacteria (known to help cause ulcers) are present.

SEE YOUR DOCTOR IF...

- Symptoms persist despite home treatments.
- *Urgently* if you bring up bright red blood or notice 'coffee grounds' in vomit or black 'tarry' stools – a bleeding ulcer may be responsible.
- You experience unexplained weight loss of 3 kilos (7 lbs) or more, jaundice or pain spreading into your back – their cause must be traced.

■ Inguinal Hernia

You may feel something 'give' in your groin (the crease between your lower abdomen and upper thigh), while heaving furniture or lifting a heavy weight. Or perhaps you have noticed a bulge or swelling. This is an inguinal hernia or 'rupture'. A small weak spot is created in the abdominal wall by the testicles when they move to the outside of the body from within the abdomen during development in the womb and the bulge is a coil of bowel protruding outwards from the abdomen's interior to just below the skin, where it can be seen and felt, especially when you *cough*.

If the muscles pinch the herniated bowel loop passing through them, they can obstruct its blood supply and the onward passage of food and waste. Signs that your hernia has become 'strangulated' in this way can include redness, swelling and intense pain, nausea and vomiting. Prompt surgery is needed to remove the damaged segment of bowel and prevent gangrene.

WHAT YOU CAN DO

- Lose excess weight – a heavy abdomen strains the muscular wall, increasing the risks of a hernia.

- Eat healthily and drink six to eight glasses of water daily to prevent or treat *constipation* – straining raises the pressure in the abdomen, which in turn increases the pressure on weak spots in the abdominal wall.

- Avoid moving furniture or lifting other heavy weights if you are unfit. Learn to lift by bending your knees, minimizing the strain on vulnerable areas.

- Take gentle regular exercise four to five times a week to increase your fitness level and learn some simple exercises to strengthen your abdominal muscles.

- Give up smoking and treat a chronic *cough* with home remedies. Seek medical help for a persistent *cough*.

- Homoeopathic remedies to take 4 times a day for 14 days while awaiting surgery:

  o Remedy of first resort – Nux vomica 6c

  o For a hernia on the right side of your groin accompanied by a cutting pain – Aesculus 6c

- Sip a soothing herbal tea to aid digestion and quell symptoms. Chamomile, peppermint and valerian are all good choices. Ask a medical herbalist about a remedy said specifically to target hernias, named 'rupturewort' (*Herniari glabra*).

- Ensure that you derive maximum benefits from your diet and calm irritability and tension, which aggravate hernia discomfort.

- *Acupressure* cannot physically reduce a hernia, but it can tone and energize the digestive organs. Good points on which to work include:

  o Crooked Pond

○ Elegant Mansion – combats anxiety, breathing difficulties, *asthma* and a chronic *cough*.

○ Three Mile Point

• Practise *relaxation* daily. This will encourage you to stop smoking, shed excess weight, take regular exercise and eat more healthily. Gentle *Yoga* (check your fitness with your doctor first) can build up the muscular strength in your abdominal wall. Beneficial asanas include the Locust, Mountain, Uddiyana and Yoga Mudra.

Drug remedies

○ Medical treatments for *cough* and *constipation*.

○ An anti-spasmodic such as mebeverine may help the shooting pains in a hernia while awaiting an operation. (Nausea and vomiting would be treated in hospital before surgery was undertaken.)

○ Analgesics (painkillers) that work without causing *constipation* as a side-effect – paracetamol, aspirin and NSAIDs (non-steroidal anti-inflammatory drugs) such as ibuprofen, naproxen.

SEE YOUR DOCTOR IF...

• You develop a lump in your groin – the diagnosis of a hernia has to be confirmed.
• The hernia increases in size or tenderness, despite home treatments.
• You develop any of the symptoms of strangulation (SEE *page 101*).

▪ Intestinal Thrush

When intestinal thrush was first recognized in the 1970s, it was believed to cause a range of health problems including *cystitis*, prostatitis (prostate gland inflammation), alcohol cravings, *depression* and persistent ringworm. Your experience of it probably includes *diarrhoea*, lots of flatulence (*wind*), especially after eating starch, fatigue, food sensitivities and vaginal thrush.

The thrush fungus, *Candida*, is a normal inhabitant of the intestine and vagina. Problems start when it becomes more active than usual, for example when your immune system is weakened by illness or stress. Antibiotics which destroy the useful bacteria that normally control *Candida* can also be responsible. The *Candida* cells then grow and penetrate the gut wall, allowing yeast by-products and undigested food particles into the bloodstream. These 'foreign bodies' are said to cause a wide range of allergic symptoms, including chronic fatigue syndrome (*myalgic encephalomyelitis, ME*) and mental and emotional problems.

WHAT YOU CAN DO

- If you have to take antibiotics, also take probiotic yoghurts and drinks to reinforce your intestines' friendly bacteria.

- Oral contraceptives and steroid drugs can also favour the spread of *Candida*. Include probiotics in your daily diet and strengthen your immune system with a wholefood diet and regular exercise.

- Refined starches and sugars are *Candida*'s natural food. Avoid these, and all items based on fermentation (for example alcohol) or containing mould (for example certain cheeses, mushrooms). Avoid fruit for the first six to eight weeks because of its sugar content. Fresh vegetables and their juices, lean sources of protein, pulses and wholegrains such as brown rice and wholewheat are all healthy choices.

- Some health experts recommend a daily supplement of *Lactobacillus acidophilus* (useful bacteria). Suitable choices exist if you are allergic to dairy products. Doses vary (and you should follow the package instructions), but one regimen prescribes 1 g daily for the first fortnight followed by 500 mg daily for 6 months.

- The B vitamin biotin is also very helpful in thrush control. Take a recommended dose daily for 2–3 months.

- Olive oil is said to help in a similar fashion to biotin. Take 20 ml (1–2 dsp) of the cold-pressed variety. Taking this neat, or flavoured with garlic or cider vinegar, for example, may give you *diarrhoea*. It is easier to include the olive oil in a salad dressing or mayonnaise and take the full amount over the course of each day.

- Try fresh garlic – not a problem if you happen to enjoy it raw. Eat several large cloves daily, or take four to six odourless garlic capsules.

- Arginine supplements are often recommended to boost the immune system when intestinal thrush is present. Therapeutic doses of amino acids are unsuitable for anyone suffering from schizophrenia or herpes (*cold sores*) and in any case are best taken under the professional guidance of a nutritionist. They may also recommend you take a gram of natural vitamin C daily and 100 mg zinc orotate in addition to a multivitamin/mineral daily supplement.

- Combat *depression*, longstanding *anxiety* or similar stress with counselling, or practise deep *relaxation, Yoga* and/or *autohypnosis*.

Drug remedies

○ Anti-fungal oral drugs such as nystatin and amphotericin are prescribed.

SEE YOUR DOCTOR IF...

- You suspect you may be suffering from intestinal thrush.
- You experience recurrent attacks of *cystitis*, vaginal thrush infections, prostate gland inflammation or the symptoms of *ME*.
- Home measures do not bring relief.

▪ Irritable Bowel Syndrome

If you suffer from irritable bowel syndrome (IBS), you will have bouts of *diarrhoea* alternating with *constipation*, as well as spells when your bowels are regular. You will get occasional cramping pains in the lower abdomen, and passing stools may hurt. You will experience annoying, uncomfortable tummy bloating and possibly a rumbling stomach, mucusy stools and *wind*. IBS can appear at any age from childhood onwards, but it is found most often between the ages of 20 and 50 years.

You are twice as likely to have IBS if you are a woman, and both dietary and psychological factors act as triggers. Highly spiced food, onions, brassicas (for example cabbage, Brussels sprouts), beer, orange juice, molasses and strong coffee can all irritate your bowel, as can a low-fibre diet or food intolerance, for example to wheat, corn, dairy products, citrus fruit and other foods. Stress factors are also important, and many people with IBS tend to be rigid, disciplined, over-conscientious, hypersensitive and prone to guilty feelings.

WHAT YOU CAN DO

- Avoid foods and other irritants to which you are sensitive.

- Drink six to eight glasses of water a day and adjust your diet to your personal needs. If fibre irritates your bowel during an attack, drink freshly squeezed vegetable and fruit juices and milky drinks, and eat milk puddings and egg dishes, minced poultry and lightly cooked fish.

- If your irritable bowel craves extra fibre, follow a wholefood diet with lots of low GI fruit and vegetables.

- Relieve bowel spasm with fennel or peppermint tea, or caraway tea made from the pounded seeds. Lie down and massage your abdomen using one or more of these oils.

- For *constipation*, suck a few comforting liquorice toffees (brush your teeth well afterwards!)

- Deep *relaxation*, *Yoga* and *autohypnosis* offer helpful relief from nagging *anxiety* and stress.

- Try a suitable *Bach Flower Remedy*. Rock Water alleviates rigid self-discipline, repression and self-denial, Beech works on intolerance and anger, and Chicory on self-pity and destructive possessiveness.

- Try these homoeopathic remedies – 4 times daily for up to 14 days:

  o For watery stools, griping tummy pain and nausea worsened by the smell of cooking: Colchicum 6c

  o For *diarrhoea* alternating with *constipation*, lots of *wind*, mucousy motions, pain in upper abdomen, and tense and anxious feelings: Argentum nit. 6c

○ For searing tummy pains, thirst, nausea, vomiting and *cystitis*: Cantharis 6c

○ For severe *abdominal pain* somewhat relieved by curling up on your side and by rubbing the troublesome area, triggered by anger: Colocynth 6c

Drug remedies

○ Anti-spasmodics such as hyoscine tablets or mebeverine hydrochloride + ispaghula husks. The latter relieves gut spasm and provides a bulking agent (SEE *Constipation*). Developed for the treatment of IBS, it comes in sachets of granules.

○ For trapped *wind* and painful bowel spasms, take peppermint oil capsules.

○ For loose watery stools, SEE *Diarrhoea*.

○ An antidepressant such as amitriptyline can be effective, especially when taken alongside an anti-spasmodic and a bulking agent.

SEE YOUR DOCTOR IF...

• You have recently developed IBS symptoms. The cause for a change of bowel habit must be established.
• You are losing weight unexpectedly.
• You notice blood in your motions.
• Home treatments do not help.

▪ Loss of Appetite

If you are trying to lose weight, you may sometimes wish that you could lose your appetite, but medically significant appetite loss (anorexia) can be life-threatening. *Anorexia nervosa,* the eating disorder linked to slimming, is most common among teenagers, while plain anorexia affects all ages. Most digestive tract disorders reduce the appetite, as do *colds* and *flu, sore throat,* liver complaints, *anxiety, depression* and physical injury. Persistent anorexia is a rare early symptom of stomach cancer.

Many drugs and chemotherapy and radiotherapy can put you off your food. Dietary deficiency of iron, zinc, folic acid, vitamin B1 and biotin can have a similar effect.

WHAT YOU CAN DO

- Take regular exercise and stop smoking.

- Take a multivitamin/mineral/trace element supplement.

- Snacking, racing through or skipping meals can interfere with your appestat mechanism. This midbrain centre prompts you to eat when required and to stop when you've had enough. Overriding its signals can dull the appetite's sensitivity, so that hunger fails to appear when the body needs food.

- Make time for three regular meals daily, plus snacks in between.

- Sit down to eat! Start with small helpings – two chopped, ripe strawberries and 15 ml (1 tbsp) of live yoghurt or a glass of freshly squeezed orange juice blended with a banana and a pinch of anise should appeal.

- Herbal teas of anise, fennel or clove all boost the appetite.

- Herbal bitters, a traditional appetite stimulant, are available in healthfood shops and pharmacies. Add a few drops to water or fruit juice, or follow the packet directions. Angostura bitters (from good off-licences) work similarly – try a couple of drops in tomato juice or iced mineral water.

- Homoeopathic remedies for appetite loss, to be taken every 8 hours for up to 2 weeks, provided this problem is not due to drugs, a diagnosed illness, food or alcohol bingeing or anorexia nervosa:

    ○ For someone who is not thirsty and is particularly put off their food by the thought of eggs or greasy food: Pulsatilla 30c

    ○ When a person is put off food by a bitter taste in the mouth, has a yellow-coated tongue and feels as though they have a hangover: Nux 30c

    ○ When appetite loss is due to grief, when a person has no interest whatever in food (although is not averse to it): Ignatia 30c

    ○ When a person is hungry but feels full up after a mouthful or two and has *wind* in the stomach: Lycopodium 30c

    ○ A specific homoeopathic remedy to be taken after an illness when a person feels in need of a tonic: Gentiana 3c. Take 5 drops half an hour before meals for 12 days.

Drug remedies

○ There are no specific drugs prescribed to stimulate appetite.

○ Drugs that cause a bad taste in the mouth and reduce appetite can sometimes be replaced with another lacking this effect.

○ Multivitamin/mineral supplements and meal replacements are widely prescribed for elderly people, convalescents and others with poor appetite.

SEE YOUR DOCTOR IF...

- Your appetite disappears for a fortnight or longer when you are in good health, or for a shorter period if you are recovering from an illness or accident.

■ Mouth Ulcers

Known medically as aphthous ulcers, these are smallish craters with a white base surrounded by a red ring of inflamed tissue. They can appear singly or in groups under or along the edge of the tongue, at the tongue's root, on the cheek linings or on the roof of the mouth. They can be very painful, especially when they occur in high friction areas where they are aggravated by talking and chewing.

Possible causes include a viral infection, certain foods (in susceptible people), stomach or bowel disturbances, fever and stress. Multiple large ulcers (up to 1½ cm/¾ inch diameter) accompanied by other symptoms such as anaemia and unexplained bruising, also occur in leukaemia and other blood disorders.

WHAT YOU CAN DO

- Oral hygiene is important. Make sure you brush your teeth at least twice daily and floss regularly.

- Minimize pain with food that doesn't require much chewing. Avoid sharp, rough foods like toast, biscuits and crisps, nuts and seeds, and eat comforting, soft and preferably warm foods such as rice pudding, milky drinks, porridge, boiled or scrambled eggs and puréed or juiced fresh vegetables and non-citrus fruit.

- Rinse your mouth regularly with warm salty water, a herbal mouthwash or freshly prepared cabbage juice (SEE *Sore Mouth or Tongue*).

- Dab ulcers with tincture of myrrh, an old remedy still sold by many pharmacists. The intense bitterness can 'draw' your mouth, but it provides great pain relief.

- Boost your immunity with a diet rich in essential nutrients, especially beta carotene (pro-vitamin A) and vitamin C, both found in fresh fruit and vegetables, and riboflavin (vitamin B2), found in green leafy vegetables, eggs, fish, kidney, liver and milk. If necessary, top up with a multivitamin and mineral supplement for a month or two.

- Vitamin E has been prescribed to treat mouth ulcers. Wheatgerm, soya beans, enriched cereals and flour, eggs and green leafy vegetables such as broccoli, spinach and Brussels sprouts are all rich sources.

- Homoeopathic remedies help many mouth ulcer sufferers. Take four times daily for up to five days:

  - For burning, stinging ulcers mainly on the tongue, aggravated by chewing food, with more saliva than usual, a coated, trembly tongue, *bad breath* and loose teeth: Mercurius 6c

  - For ulcers soothed by warm water, and a dry and burning mouth: Arsenicum 6c

  - For ulcers that bleed when touched or after eating, a hot and tender mouth and possibly oral thrush: Borax 6c

- Combat stress with regular *relaxation* and *Yoga*, and ensure sound sleep (SEE *Snoring and Sleep Apnoea*).

Drug remedies

○ Use an antiseptic, steroid or anaesthetic mouthwash, spray or paste/gel (SEE *Sore Mouth or Tongue*).

○ Take two paracetamol or an anti-inflammatory medicine such as ibuprofen to relieve pain and stinging.

SEE YOUR DOCTOR IF...

- Home remedies do not help.
- You feel generally unwell and run down.
- You need help such as counselling to deal with emotional stress.

■ Piles

Piles, also known as haemorrhoids, are small red tender swellings in and around the back passage or anus. They can be external – visible all the time – or internal – descending when you open your bowels, then retreating back into the anus. Symptoms include pain on passing motions and blood on the lavatory paper, on the surface of the stools or on your clothing. Your back passage may feel itchy, prickly and sore (SEE *Anal Itching*).

Piles develop from small anal and rectal veins, which like those in the leg, become varicosed when undue strain is placed upon them.

Often running in families, piles are triggered by a build-up of pressure inside your abdomen. This can happen when you are very overweight, pregnant, have a chronic (for example a smoker's) *cough*, have to strain when you go the lavatory or frequently lift heavy objects and the delicate anal and rectal veins become overstretched, forming piles. The risks of developing them increases if you eat too little fibre and rarely exercise.

WHAT YOU CAN DO

- Take more exercise and lose surplus weight.

- Watch your weight gain during pregnancy.

- Avoid dehydration and straining to pass hard motions. Follow the nutritional advice and home remedies for *constipation*. Blueberries are said to aid piles sufferers.

- Stop smoking.

- Take home remedies or seek medical treatment for a troublesome *cough*.

- Avoid sitting on very hot or cold surfaces, such as radiators and the ground outside in winter – both encourage piles.

- Relieve inflamed piles by cutting out coffee, chocolate, cocoa, highly spiced dishes and cola drinks, or eliminate one at a time and observe the effect.

- Keep your drinking within safe limits. Excessive alcohol breakdown products present in the motions irritate the anus and aggravate piles.

- Medical herbalists may recommend bathing piles with an infusion of fresh chervil.

- For a tried and tested folk remedy, chop up and boil several leeks, strain and freeze the water into ice cubes. Apply to stinging piles for immediate relief.

- Dab piles with witch hazel solution or cream night and morning and after opening your bowels.

- Homoeopathic remedies – to be taken four times daily for up to five days:

  o For bleeding, when the anus feels bruised and sore: Hamamelis 6c

  o For great itching, frequent bleeding, *constipation* and a desire to open the bowels: Collinsonia 6c

  o You can also dab piles with Hamamelis solution or use peony ointment suppositories (stocked by homoeopathic pharmacies).

- The *Yoga* asanas Fish, Plough and Shoulder Stand can all prove helpful.

Drug remedies

o Bulking agents such as ispaghula husks are kinder to piles than osmotic or irritant laxatives (SEE *Constipation*).

o Anti-inflammatory, antiseptic and local anaesthetic medication all ease bowel opening when piles are present. Most are available as creams, ointments and suppositories which you insert into the back passage.

SEE YOUR DOCTOR IF...

- You have bleeding from the back passage. Note whether the blood is bright red (i.e. coming from the anus or rectum) and on the motions (probably piles) or mixed in with them (some other cause). *Never assume that piles are responsible for anal bleeding – the cause must be identified.*
- Simple home treatments fail to help.

■ Sore Mouth or Tongue

A sore mouth or tongue interferes with eating and talking, and can make you feel wretched. Common causes include scalding or heavily spiced foods and drinks, jagged teeth or ill-fitting dentures, *mouth ulcers* and thrush (a fungal infection).

Boiling foods and drinks, concentrated vinegar, mustard, chilli or similar spices, strong bitter chocolate and very strong cheddar cheese can all destroy patches of the mouth's lining. Dead bits of 'skin' come away as small white fragments, leaving sore areas behind. Certain drugs, such as the anticonvulsant phenytoin, can also make your mouth sore. Broken teeth and dentures scratch and tear the tongue or inner cheek, producing painful wounds sometimes mistaken for *mouth ulcers*.

Oral thrush tends to affect elderly, diabetic or severely ill people, denture wearers, asthmatics and newborn babies. It can also follow a course of antibiotics or steroids and appears in white curd-like patches revealing red-raw flesh when scraped away.

WHAT YOU CAN DO

- Avoid obvious dietary irritants (the habitual consumption of highly spiced or scalding foods or drinks has also been linked to mouth and gullet cancer).

- To soothe the pain of a burn or irritation due to spices or acidic food, take a mouthful of cold water and hold it for a minute or two before swallowing. Alternatively, suck an ice cube. The pain will return, but you will obtain immediate relief.

- See a dentist as soon as possible when a broken tooth or dentures are causing trouble.

- Wash out your mouth with a dilute solution of TCP or buy a *mouth ulcer* remedy and apply it every three hours to sore areas not caused by thrush.

- *Gently* swab patches of thrush with a 3 per cent solution of hydrogen peroxide mixed with an equal volume of warm salt water.

- Check your diet. Thrush tends to set in when your immune system is depleted, so top up your vitamin and mineral intake with lots of raw or lightly cooked vegetables and fruit, including blueberries and their freshly squeezed juices. (Avoid citrus fruit because their acids will sting.)

- Juice a cabbage and swill a little round your mouth, bathing the painful area, swallow and repeat. Cabbages supply a factor (termed vitamin U) which soothes inflamed digestive tract membranes.

- Use a herbal mouthwash three to four times daily. Neat aloe vera juice is excellent for burns and inflammation. Alternatively, dilute liquid echinacea with tepid water.

- An *aromatherapy* mouthwash using tea tree oil dispersed in tepid water reduces inflammation and fights infection.

Drug remedies

- A couple of paracetamol or an anti-inflammatory such as nurofen will relieve sore mouth misery for a few hours.

- Anti-inflammatory rinses or mouth sprays containing benzydamine relieve oral soreness and inflammation.

- A low dose of the steroid triamcinolone in the form of a paste eases mouth soreness and injury.

- Oral gels and sprays containing anaesthetic temporarily numb mouth pain.

SEE YOUR DOCTOR IF...

- You have thrush. An anti-fungal liquid or pastilles available on prescription can cure the infection.
- You take phenytoin and/or suspect that this (or any other medication) is making your mouth sore.
- Any persistent mouth problem fails to disappear despite simple measures. Anaemia and other blood disorders can cause mouth and tongue soreness, as can a poor diet.

▪ Stomach Upset

Feeling sick (nausea) and being sick (vomiting) often follow a food or alcohol binge, but sometimes these symptoms start out of the blue. Gastroenteritis due to food or drink contaminated by a virus or *E. coli* bacteria from the large bowel is usually responsible. Besides vomiting, you may feel faint and exhausted, have cramping tummy pains, fever and *diarrhoea*, and continue to retch long after your stomach is empty.

For other causes of nausea and vomiting, see Anxiety, Gall Bladder Inflammation, Headache/Migraine, Heartburn/Indigestion and Motion Sickness.

WHAT YOU CAN DO

- Avoid bingeing on rich foods. Line your stomach with a glass of milk and a sandwich before an evening's drinking and aim to keep your alcohol intake within sensible limits.

- Evening primrose oil can both help prevent and relieve a hangover – take 4 × 500 mg capsules with water.

- Wash your hands and keep work surfaces, cooking utensils, dish and tea cloths scrupulously clean.

- Follow the advice for safe food storage suggested by fridge manufacturers and others.

- Do not try to soldier on with persistent vomiting, severe *abdominal pain* and/or fever. Rest, and avoid solid food and milky drinks. Combat nausea with cinnamon, ginger or peppermint herbal tea, chew a small piece of crystallized or fresh root ginger or sip 15 ml (1 tbsp) ginger wine, either neat or diluted with warm or chilled water.

- Use one of the standard pharmaceutical remedies to replace water and electrolytes (body salts). Alternatively, stir 15 ml (1 tbsp) of glucose or sugar, 5 ml (1 tsp) salt and a good squeeze of lemon or lime juice (orange can aggravate nausea) into 500 ml (1 pint) of water. Small frequent sips will help to prevent dehydration and soothe your inflamed stomach.

- Flat Coca-Cola can help – it was originally developed as a remedy for nausea.

- To speed up recovery once vomiting has stopped, try some herbal slippery elm bark or marshmallow to reduce stomach and bowel inflammation.

- Try the following homoeopathic remedies at 15-minute (or longer) intervals, for up to 10 doses:

  ○ For nausea and vomiting due to food poisoning or peptic ulcer when there is also *diarrhoea*, warm drinks ease stomach pain and the symptoms are worst between midnight and 2 a.m.: Arsenicum 6c

  ○ For vomiting which starts 2–3 hours after eating, with painful retching, the person waking around 4 a.m., being unable to return to sleep and feeling hungover, especially after too much to eat or if a peptic ulcer is present: Nux 6c

Drug remedies

o Pharmaceutical electrolyte + glucose mixtures prepared as directed with water (these are nearly always used to treat gastroenteritis in babies and small children in preference to more potent drugs).

o Prescription drugs for vomiting include metoclopromide and prochlorperazine.

o Once you can keep fluids down, a paracetamol + codeine compound tablet can help quell tummy pains and reduce fever.

SEE YOUR DOCTOR IF...

- *Urgently* if signs of dehydration appear – a dry mouth, pallor, exhaustion and loss of skin elasticity. Dehydration can be fatal, especially in children and elderly people.
- *Urgently* if you bring up large spots of bright red blood or 'coffee grounds' vomit, as internal bleeding may be present (SEE *Heartburn/Indigestion*).
- *Urgently* if you have belching, bad-smelling vomit and a distended stomach – you may have an obstruction.
- Your symptoms are especially severe or fail to respond to home treatments.

■ Threadworms

Some people who suspect that they may have worms postpone seeking medical advice because they are ashamed of their problem. Worms, however, can infest anybody. Threadworms or pinworms are the most common variety, especially among school-children. They appear in the faeces as little white threads about 1.2 cm (½ inch) long. The adult worms inhabit the rectum (the final part of the large intestine) and the female comes out at night to lay her eggs around the anal opening. This area becomes intensely itchy and girls can experience further irritation of the vagina and/or urethra (bladder outlet tube) if the worms spread.

The larvae (immature worms) hatch out after about 6 hours, and, if swallowed, for example from fingers scratching the back passage during sleep, mature in the large bowel and continue the cycle. Eggs found in dust or dirt at home or at school also pass on the infestation if they are swallowed.

WHAT YOU CAN DO

- Keep dirt and dust to a minimum.

- Wash your hands after housework and visits to the lavatory, after playing with or grooming pets and always before eating.

- Minimize nocturnal itching with a bath or shower before bed and use one of the remedies for *anal itching*.

- Wear pyjamas to minimize the chances of scratching and swallowing eggs and larvae while asleep.

- Keep fingernails short and scrub them every day.

- Worm cat and dog pets.

- Chew two cloves of garlic a day, if liked, until the worms have cleared.

- Alternatively, drink a glass of freshly squeezed cabbage juice every morning for three mornings. This is a traditional remedy for intestinal worm infestation, with the bonus of warding off bacterial infection in parts of the bowel damaged by the worms and promoting the healing process. The flavour can be improved by the addition of fresh carrot juice.

- Ramsons (*Allium ursinum*) is a potent antiseptic herb similar to garlic. Medical herbalists may prescribe them to get rid of threadworms, either as the juice, as an infusion or possibly as an enema.

- Homoeopathic remedies – to be taken 3 times a day for up to 14 days:

  o For an itchy bottom, a child who is irritable and inclined to pick their nose, grinds their teeth, is very hungry and has dark rings under their eyes: Cina 6c

  o For an itchy bottom and itchy nose, with the irritation worse in the evening, a child who is restless in sleep and complains of a crawling sensation in their rectum after passing motions: Teucrium 6c

  o A standby remedy if the others fail: Santoninum 6c

Drug remedies

o Sachets containing piperazine, which paralyses thread-worms, and senna to ensure that the bowels open effectively (SEE *Constipation*). Packs contain two sachets to be made up with water – one for immediate use and the other for a repeat dose 14 days later. (Unsuitable for children under 3 months.)

o Tablets or suspension containing mebendazole, which immo-bilizes and kills threadworms and several other varieties of intestinal worm. Unsuitable for children under 2 years.

> **SEE YOUR DOCTOR IF...**
>
> - Threadworms do not disappear with home treatment.
> - You develop *abdominal pain*, bleeding from the back passage or similar symptoms.

■ Toothache and Sensitive Teeth

Toothache resulting from dental decay tends to be sharper than gum pain and fairly easy to trace to the tooth concerned. Decay results when the plaque-forming bacteria break down sugar molecules, releasing acid. The acid attacks the tooth's outer enamel and, if allowed to progress, reaches the underlying substance (dentine), where it breaks down calcium salts.

If conditions in your mouth remain acidic because you neglect your teeth or eat too many sugary foods, the erosion continues until it reaches the live nerve fibres in the tooth's centre or pulp. Then your tooth will become sensitive to very cold or hot foods/drinks and will start to ache.

Severe throbbing toothache may be due to an abscess (SEE *Abscesses and Boils*), caused by a build-up of pus in the tooth's pulp, where bacteria can thrive and multiply.

WHAT YOU CAN DO

- Visit your dentist! A tooth cavity cannot repair itself (although small erosions can be filled in by salts found in saliva, provided the mouth's acidic conditions are neutralized). Modern dental treatment is far less painful and exhausting than toothache, which can only worsen and may trouble you for weeks, or until the tooth falls out.

- Avoid very hot or cold foods and foods high in sugar. Boost your calcium intake with low-fat dairy foods, broccoli and other green leafy vegetables.

- Rinse your mouth with warm salty water to remove acid and stray bits of food.

- Antiseptic mouthwashes of TCP or tea tree oil in warm water are also effective.

- Examine the painful area (if accessible) using a light and mirror. Gently ease any food particles out of gaps on either side of the aching tooth. *Any* reduction in pressure in the affected area should help to ease the pain.

- Gently dab the root of the tooth with cotton wool soaked in essential oil of clove. Leave the swab in place for a few minutes if possible. The taste is intense and it may stimulate saliva flow, but it brings great relief.

- Throbbing pain and facial swelling point to an abscess. Make a hot compress with essential oil of chamomile and bind in place with a scarf.

- *Acupressure* can give temporary relief. Try massaging the following points:

  o Facial Beauty

  o Jaw Chariot

- Try these homoeopathic remedies – one dose every 5 minutes for up to ten doses:

  o For toothache with tender, spongy gums that easily bleed, loose teeth and *bad breath*: Mercurius 6c

  o For insufferable toothache aggravated by cold air, warm food and drink and coffee in the evening: Chamomilla 6c

o For bad toothache aggravated by heat and hot food and relieved by applying (wrapped) ice cubes: Coffea 6c

Drug remedies

o Two paracetamol or ibuprofen or a paracetamol/codeine combination every 4–6 hours to relieve inflammation and pain.

SEE YOUR DOCTOR IF...

- The pain is intolerable and you have to wait for an emergency dental appointment. Your doctor can prescribe stronger painkillers, and an antibiotic if your symptoms suggest a dental abscess.

■ Wind

Belching – bringing up wind through the mouth – can be caused by swallowing air when nervous, eating too quickly, over-rich foods and binge eating. Trying to repress a belch can prove painful, because its function is to reduce undue pressure within the stomach. You can inadvertently add to the problem by trying too hard to belch, thereby swallowing further air. Stomach wind is a feature of *heartburn* and *indigestion*, including hiatus hernia, and can be brought on by over-spiced dishes and by fatty food if you suffer from gallstones (SEE *Gall Bladder Inflammation*).

Back passage wind can be even more embarrassing. It's a common feature of *intestinal thrush, colitis, stomach upset, irritable bowel syndrome* and *diarrhoea*, and it is commonly caused by the bacterial fermentation of food, especially in constipated people. This can happen if you eat large quantities of sweets, chocolate and other sugary foods, or drink a lot of alcohol. Eggs, beans or peas are also best avoided if you are prone to bowel wind, because they aggravate the problem and are broken down by bowel bacteria into sulphurous gases with an unpleasant smell.

WHAT YOU CAN DO

- Try to pinpoint the underlying cause for an ongoing wind problem.

- Eat more slowly, sit down to meals and keep talking, laughing and the consumption of alcohol and other liquids to a minimum during meals.

- Avoid recognized food triggers and any foods or drinks you suspect may upset you. Starches and refined sugars are often to blame.

- If you think anxiety may be responsible, try regular *relaxation* and *Yoga* to help to beat tension and teach you to control your breathing.

- Suck a peppermint to help burping and release stomach gas.

- Suck an aniseed ball, or try aniseed tea, using the ground-up seeds to make an infusion. Sipped slowly, this combats *indigestion* caused by nervousness, promotes calm breathing and relaxation after a meal and can prevent *hiccups* and belching.

- Other carminative plants whose oils help to expel gas from the intestines and relieve the accompanying pain include basil, bergamot, caraway, chamomile, cinnamon, lemon, nutmeg and rosemary.

- Try the Knee to Chest *Yoga* asana.

- Homoeopathic remedies to take every half-hour for up to ten doses:

o If belching relieves discomfort: Carbo veg. 6c

o If belching brings no relief: China 6c

o For belching with nausea, the person feels worse in hot rooms: Pulsatilla 6c

o When there is a craving for sugary foods, a bloated tummy, *diarrhoea* and the wind is worse when the person is worrying about a future event: Argentum nit. 6c

● Try *acupressure* – Sea of Energy relieves excess gas and other digestive problems.

(SEE *also Intestinal Thrush*.)

Drug remedies

o Liquid suspensions combining an antacid such as aluminium hydroxide and a deflatulent such as activated dimeticone combat stomach acid and belching.

o Take an Alka-Seltzer or similar to settle your stomach. It will calm acidity and its fizz stimulates the release of excess gas.

o Peppermint oil capsules can help burping. Taken for *irritable bowel syndrome*, they help to prevent painful spasm and the formation of surplus bowel gas.

SEE YOUR DOCTOR IF...

● You have *indigestion*, heartburn or other symptoms that have not responded to simple home treatments.
● You believe anxiety may be causing your wind, and *relaxation*, *Yoga*, etc. have not helped.

9

Nose, Throat and Airway Ailments

● Asthma ● Bronchitis ● The common cold
● Cough ● Flu ● Hayfever ● Hiccups ● Hoarseness
and loss of voice ● Nosebleeds ● Sinusitis ● Snoring
and sleep apnoea ● Sore throat and tonsillitis

▪ Asthma

During an asthma attack your chest becomes 'tight', making you
fight for breath. You may also become a bit wheezy or short of
breath in cold weather, when upset or excited, or after moderate
exercise such as climbing a flight of stairs.

The cause, from a practical viewpoint, is the hypersensitivity of
your smaller air tubes to allergens, pollutants, infections and
stress, all of which cause constriction of the air tubes' walls. This
narrowing gives rise to the characteristic wheeze and the terrifying battle to breathe in and out. Panic narrows the airways further,
sometimes turning the sufferer pale and sweaty, with bluish lips
due to oxygen shortage.

When the linings of the bronchioles become inflamed, for example due to a chest infection or allergy, they secrete extra mucus, which narrows the airways still further. Most asthmatics have a fundamental immune system problem, known as atopy, and often suffer from related conditions, too, such as *eczema*, *hayfever* and nettle-rash (*hives*, urticaria).

WHAT YOU CAN DO

- Avoid known personal triggers where possible.

- A wholefood diet boosts immunity against both allergies and infections. Recommended juices include carrot with a little spinach, carrot and celery (any proportions), and grapefruit. Pineapple, which contains the enzyme betaine, has recently been found helpful.

- Lose excess weight and take regular exercise to tone heart and lungs.

- Cider vinegar is used with benefit by many asthma sufferers. One recipe mixes 10 ml (2 tsp) each of organic cider vinegar and runny honey with a tumbler of water, to be taken 2–3 times daily.

- Propolis, a natural bactericidal substance made by bees to keep their hives infection-free, is available as a liquid, capsules and lozenges. Take a supplement when needed, especially in the pollen season if you also suffer from *hayfever*.

- Herbal medicines prescribed to treat asthma include garlic (especially) and also aniseed, cat's claw, cowslip, elecampane, gumplant, lavender, liquorice, poppy petals and thyme. Lime- or linden-flower tea has a calming effect and also relaxes blood vessels, helping to reduce inflammation. Buy this in sachets or make an infusion yourself using fresh or dried leaves.

- Towel-over-head inhalations of essential oils of chamomile, eucalyptus or Roman chamomile all encourage the constricted bronchiolar walls to relax. You can also add a few drops to your bathwater or inhale them from a tissue or oil warmer.

- Try homoeopathic remedies every 15 minutes up to a total of ten doses:

  o For an attack that starts after exposure to a cold dry wind, especially when the person is anxious, fears death and the attack starts at night: Aconite 30c

  o For exhaustion and weakness, cold clammy skin, rattly breathing and difficulty in coughing up phlegm: Antimonium tartrate 6c

- Useful *acupressure* points include:

  o Elegant Mansion

  o Great Abyss

  o Lung Associated Point

- Practise regular *relaxation*. Useful *Yoga* asanas include the Complete Breath, Corpse, Fish, Mountain and Shoulder Stand.

Drug remedies

o Medicinal inhalers include bronchiolar relaxants, steroids to combat inflammation and others that help to prevent allergic reactions.

o *Cough* linctuses can reduce mucus secretion and night-time coughing.

o Steroids reduce inflammation in severe attacks.

o Antibiotics treat or prevent a chest infection.

SEE YOUR DOCTOR IF...

- For regular checkups.
- You develop a chest infection.
- Prescribed medications or home remedies do not help.

▪ Bronchitis

You may develop acute bronchitis following a *cold* or *flu*, when viruses spread to the lungs from your nose and throat. You develop a fever, a painful *cough* and aching muscles, and feel generally unwell. A day or so later, your *cough* starts to produce phlegm and is less troublesome.

Chronic bronchitis, a different disease, results from repeated air passage irritation by smoke, dust and other pollutants. Copious mucus forms and bacterial infections are frequent. You always have phlegm on your chest and a wet cough, and often become wheezy and short of breath. This is due to the destruction of tiny air sacs in your lungs where oxygen and carbon dioxide gases are exchanged.

WHAT YOU CAN DO

- Stay away from irritants such as cigarette smoke, noxious gases and other pollutants, and, where possible, avoid cold weather, icy winds and getting cold and wet for long periods.

- For acute bronchitis, stay in bed, drink lots of fluid and take two paracetamol, aspirin or ibuprofen three times daily. Watch out for a fever and coloured phlegm.

- Towel-over-head steam inhalations help to clear thick mucus. Add benzoin (the active ingredient in Friar's balsam), eucalyptus, hyssop, menthol, peppermint or tea tree essential oils. Rub your chest with 20 ml (4 tsp) almond oil mixed with 10 drops thyme oil and/or any of the above oils.

- Herbal remedies for bronchitis often contain cowslip, elecampane, thyme, white horehound and/or valerian. Ask your pharmacist to recommend a good herbal *cough* mixture.

- Try to eat some raw garlic daily to ward off infection. You can also mash garlic with some Vaseline and rub this on your chest, or crush a couple of cloves and eat mixed with a tablespoon of runny organic honey. This sounds disgusting but is, in fact, delicious.

- *Acupressure* – try the following points:

  o Ding Chuan

  o Elegant Mansion

  o Heaven Rushing Out (specifically recommended for bronchitis)

  o Heavenly Pillar

Chronic bronchitis

- Consider changing your diet (if necessary) to include more fresh fruit and vegetables, plus their freshly squeezed juices. Cut down radically on junk food high in saturated animal fat and refined sugar and take a multivitamin and mineral supplement daily, with extra infection-fighting zinc, Siberian ginseng and B complex to counterbalance stress. Vitamin C with bioflavonoids is another potent immune-system booster and, like vitamin A, helps to repair damaged membrane linings, for example in your nose, throat and air passages.

- It is absolutely vital that you stop smoking. Use patches or chewing gum to curb nicotine cravings, or chew sunflower seeds which do this naturally.

- Try acupuncture to strengthen your immunity and subdue nicotine cravings.

Drug remedies

○ Cough linctuses, as for *Cough*.

○ Pseudoephedrine medications to control mucus production.

○ Karvol capsules to clear air passages (dissolve in hot water and inhale).

○ Inhalers prescribed by your doctor to expand narrowed air tubes, for example salbutamol or a steroid type to combat inflammation.

○ Antibiotics prescribed by your GP if secondary bacterial infection sets in.

○ Nicotine patches or chewing gum to help you stop smoking.

SEE YOUR DOCTOR IF...

- You have chronic bronchitis.
- You have a fever and yellow/green phlegm and/or a painful cough.
- Any of your symptoms worsen or fail to respond to home treatments.

■ The Common Cold

Between them, colds and *flu* are responsible for more lost working days throughout the world than any other disorder, including backache. Heavy colds are often mistaken for *flu*, although the two illnesses are distinct. We tend to catch colds during the autumn and winter – not because of cold wet weather, as often supposed, but because we are more likely to be in a crowded, stuffy, enclosed environment at work or at home, where windows remain closed, warm air is recycled and we inhale other people's germs.

Several hundred different species of cold virus exist, all of which cause the familiar shivery feeling, sneezing and running nose. You may also develop a *sore throat* and *cough* and find your nose becomes stuffy with thick coloured catarrh after the initial 'wet' phase. You should get over a mild cold in a few days; more severe ones can last a week or longer.

WHAT YOU CAN DO

- There is no cure for a cold, but you can reduce your chances of catching one (or passing one on) by remembering that it's highly infectious and transmitted in germ-laden nasal and throat secretions when we sneeze and *cough*. Use clean tissues freely, keep them away from other people and burn or otherwise dispose of them sensibly.

- Boost your resistance with a healthy diet and *relaxation*, fresh air and exercise.

- Go to bed if you feel really ill and/or have a fever. Drink lots of fluid – water (mineral or tap), fruit and vegetable juices – and eat antioxidant-rich blueberries, fresh garlic, oranges and broccoli or drink their juices. Herbal teas such as green tea soothe inflamed membranes and boost your immunity, chamomile tea helps if you are anxious and fretful (about all the jobs you are leaving to others!) Two paracetamol or ibuprofen two to three times daily will make you feel more comfortable.

- Zinc supplements have been shown to relieve colds and *sore throats*. Turkey and oats are rich sources of zinc.

- To relieve general cold symptoms, sip hot elderflower tea, which you can make using fresh or dried flowers (from a healthfood shop).

- To relieve nasal stuffiness and catarrh, inhale essences of benzoin, eucalyptus, lavender, lemon, pine and/or thyme, either from capsules available from pharmacists, used as directed, or in the steam of boiling water to which you have added a few drops of the essential oil(s).

Drug remedies

○ Take 2 paracetamol or ibuprofen every 3–4 hours as needed up to 8 daily.

○ Alternatively, use any of the cold preparations to relieve feverishness and congestion from your pharmacist.

○ Gargle with any standard antiseptic throat preparation your pharmacist recommends.

○ Suck throat lozenges, for example honey and lemon, blackcurrant or cherry.

○ Rub comforting Vicks on your chest to aid breathing.

SEE YOUR DOCTOR IF...

- Your cold worsens or is not relieved by home measures.
- You develop a painfully *sore throat,* high fever, persistent *cough* with green or yellow phlegm, earache or other worrying symptoms.

▪ Cough

A perfectly timed cough is a social asset, but symptomatic coughing can be painful and exhausting. Chemical or physical irritants can all be responsible. A dry repetitive cough is typically due either to an upper airway infection (SEE *Sore Throat*) or irritation by smoke, noxious fumes, mucus, blood, pus or (rarely) a tumour. A post-nasal drip can cause a wet or dry cough.

Lung infections tend to produce a wet cough, with yellow or green-coloured phlegm when bacteria are responsible. A few small streaks of blood can appear during a violent cough, due to small blood vessel damage.

Long-standing conditions such as *asthma*, chronic *bronchitis* and emphysema all produce characteristic coughs with, perhaps, wheezing, breathlessness and blue-tinged mucous membranes when insufficient oxygen is being taken into the lungs.

WHAT YOU CAN DO

- Avoid airborne irritants as far as possible.

- Check whether a chicken or fish bone might have lodged in your throat (this can cause violent or persistent coughing) (SEE *Choking*, under *First Aid*).

- Treat *colds, flu* and *sore throats* with home remedies.

- Check your temperature and inspect any coughed-up phlegm – you may need to see a doctor if symptoms persist (SEE *Bronchitis*).

- Vigorous coughing can cause vomiting, through its mechanical effects on your stomach muscles. Try taking frequent small sips of liquid and small readily digested meals that will soon pass from your stomach.

- Herbal remedies for coughs:

  o Mix 30 ml (2 tbsp) of raspberry vinegar, preferably organic, with the same quantity of runny clover or other organic honey. Sip 10 ml (2 tsp) at bedtime or whenever a dry cough strikes.

  o Valerian herbal remedies can be powerful expectorants (aid in bringing up phlegm).

  o For night-time coughing, a glass of hot strong black-currant drink works well, or try 15 ml (1tbsp) of freshly made blackcurrant jelly or jam mixed with the same quantity of very hot water. This is both delicious and soothing.

- *Acupressure* – try these points:

  o Ding Chuan

  o Heavenly Pillar – this helps to relieve a *sore throat* giving rise to coughing

  o Vital Diaphragm

Drug remedies

o Decongestant medicines containing pseudoephedrine reduce the amount of mucus produced by the nose, and therefore a post-nasal drip.

o Expectorant cough linctuses increase the volume but decrease the stickiness of phlegm, making it easier to cough up.

o Cough medicines such as pholcodine and codeine linctus act on the brain's cough centre, suppressing a tiring cough.

SEE YOUR DOCTOR IF...

- Your cough lasts for longer than 2 weeks despite home treatment.
- You have a fever and produce yellow or green phlegm – you may need an antibiotic.
- You notice a stabbing knife-like pain when you cough.
- You cough up blood.

■ Flu

Influenza, which may start as a *cold*, soon produces the telltale muscular aches in the legs, arms and back, a throbbing *headache*, fever and often a painful *cough*. It is passed on in the same way as a *cold*, but it can prove harder to shake off. It kills thousands of people every year, especially elderly people, small children and others with chronic illnesses that make them vulnerable. Flu vaccinations are normally available in the autumn to high-risk groups and it is sometimes possible to pay for the vaccination if you do not qualify for free treatment.

Flu can cause *heavy perspiration*, so you are more at risk from dehydration than you are with a *cold*. This is largely responsible for flu's most unpleasant symptoms, especially the 'ill' feeling, *headache* and aching limbs.

WHAT YOU CAN DO

- Retire to bed as soon as the symptoms set in. Check your temperature every few hours and preferably avoid solid food while feverish. Take a warm shower or bath to relieve aching muscles, particularly if you are perspiring heavily.

- Remember that you need to convalesce from flu and cannot simply return to full activities on your first day up. Keep meals small at first and reintroduce exercise gradually. Eat several cloves of fresh garlic daily if you can, or take garlic capsules.

- Use the *cold* remedies mentioned above, as required.

- Sip cool water frequently, or make up your own bedside drink: to 450 ml (1 pint) of water, add a teaspoonful of salt, a tablespoonful of powdered glucose or sugar, and the juice of a grapefruit, lemon, lime and/or orange. Grate in some zest for extra flavour and add a bit of the pith which is rich in bioflavonoids, the powerful antioxidant found in nature with vitamin C. Stir and sip heated or with ice cubes.

- Soothe a throbbing *headache* with a cold compress: add a few drops of lavender, melissa or rosemary essential oil to a small basin of cold/chilled water. Fold a clean towel or headscarf into a bandanna, saturate and bind round your forehead.

- Sip herbal teas recommended for flu symptoms, such as chamomile, hyssop and thyme. Take some echinacea, fresh raspberries and/or Siberian ginseng to boost your immunity. Ease aching muscles by adding a few drops of essential oils of aspic, black pepper, mandarin, neroli or petitgrain to a warm bath or add according to package directions to carrier oil, stroke gently into your muscles, relax for an hour then take a warm shower.

- Try these homoeopathic remedies every 2 hours for up to 10 doses:

  o For symptoms that come on suddenly, very high temperature, mild delirium, staring eyes and a flushed face: Belladonna 30c

○ For severe pains in limbs as though broken, bursting head, shivering, sore eyeballs: Eupatorium 6c

○ For eyes and nose hot and streaming, chills, exhaustion, wants frequent sips of water: Arsenicum 6c

Watch out for post-viral blues – flu can be physically and emotionally depleting (SEE *Depression*). Useful asanas include the Corpse, Mountain, Posterior Stretch and Shoulder Stand. Soothe headaches with the Corpse, Neck and Eye Exercises and Shoulder Roll.

Drug remedies

○ Vaccination greatly reduces your chances of contracting flu.

○ Paracetamol, aspirin or an anti-inflammatory such as ibuprofen three to four times daily while aching muscles and fever last.

○ Antibiotics to prevent or treat a bacterial throat or chest infection (common complications).

SEE YOUR DOCTOR IF...

• You are worried by a high fever, aching muscles and joints, painful throat or other symptoms.
• Simple home measures do not bring relief.
• Post-viral blues turn into *depression* which you cannot shake off.

▪ Hayfever

'Hayfever' is a misnomer because it doesn't make you feverish, nor is it caused by hay! Your immune system misinterprets harmless pollen and fungal spores as threatening and makes antibodies against them, releasing histamine. This triggers the familiar nasal prickling and tingling, the 'sniffles' and persistent sneezing. A stuffy nose follows and your eyes water, itch and become bloodshot. The roof of your mouth and your ears can irritate, too.

Persistent, severe hayfever can lead to chronic *sinusitis*, ear infections and nasal polyps – swellings in the nose which obstruct breathing. Attacks usually start in your teens and twenties. You run an increased risk of hayfever attacks if you or close family members suffer from other allergic complaints such as *eczema*, *asthma* or nettle-rash (SEE *Hives*).

WHAT YOU CAN DO

Prevention

- Keep track of the pollen count, announced daily in spring and summer during radio and television weather slots.

- Stay indoors if possible when the pollen count is high.

- Avoid obvious trouble spots such as parks, gardens and meadows.

- Keep air vents and windows closed, especially in the bedroom – if feasible, choose your next car with an integral pollen filter.

- Mow the lawn, weed flowerbeds, etc., before 7 a.m. or after 7 p.m. – or delegate to others!

- Shower every evening to remove pollen grains from skin and hair.

- Protect your eyes with wraparound shades. Don't rub them if they itch.

- Buy and use an air ionizer, a small machine which sucks in the surrounding air, and expels it in a fresher, purer form rich in negatively charged air particles (ions). Negative ions combat free radical production due to atmospheric pollution, kill airborne germs and promote healthy airways and lungs.

Remedies

- Oranges, blueberries, broccoli and garlic all boost immunity. Organic honey, particularly comb honey, contains pollen granules which, paradoxically, help to relieve hayfever symptoms. Many hayfever sufferers find pollen capsules and royal jelly (a bee product) helpful, too.

- Keep dairy products to a minimum – they increase mucus formation in your nose and throat.

- Useful supplements include natural vitamin C, with bioflavonoids for its antihistamine effects, and anti-stress high potency vitamin B complex, with extra calcium pantothenate and pyridoxine (vitamin B6) for severe symptoms.

- Rosehip tea (or wine) is a traditional hayfever remedy. Try any of the *sinusitis* remedies for a blocked nose. Some sufferers boil a handful of fresh or dried eucalyptus leaves, strain and spray around the house and round their bedroom nightly.

- Try these homoeopathic remedies as often as necessary for up to ten doses:

  o For sneezing, a 'peppery' nose' without thick discharge and itchy ears and palate, especially when occurring early in the season: Arundo 6c

  o For persistent sneezing and heavy, watering eyes combined with lethargy, dizziness and a shaky feeling: Gelsemium 6c

  o If you are exhausted but restless with the hayfever, have a slight temperature, a tight chest and burning throat and feel better in warm surroundings: Arsenicum 6c

Drug remedies

○ Antihistamines – start taking tablets 3–4 weeks before symptoms are due. Fexofenadine and descloratidine cause minimal (or no) drowsiness.

○ Nasal sprays include azolastine, excellent for sneezing and a streaming nose.

○ Eye drops, for example ketotifen, soothe irritated, inflamed eyes.

○ Steroidal nasal sprays, for example beclometasone, or non-steroidal sprays with sodium cromoglycate are useful for persistent stuffiness.

SEE YOUR DOCTOR IF...

- If you get wheezy or short of breath on high pollen count days.
- You wish to discuss skin testing and desensitizing injections against specific pollens.

▪ Hiccups

Pope Pius XII died of intractable hiccups in the 1950s. Generally, however, hiccups are a harmless, if irritating, phenomenon caused by irritation of the phrenic nerve supplying the muscles of the diaphragm. The diaphragm goes briefly into spasm, sucking air rapidly down the windpipe. But the indrawn breath is stopped in its tracks by the sudden snapping shut of the glottis (chamber containing the vocal cords, between the back of the throat and the main passageway to the lungs). This causes the characteristic 'hic' sound.

The cause of common or garden hiccups is often impossible to pinpoint, although triggers include too much food or alcohol, eating or drinking 'on the run', carbonated drinks, hot spicy food, irritating fumes, cold air or water, a sudden fright or shock, nervousness and trying to suppress an overwhelming urge to laugh.

Rarely, hiccups can result from drugs such as muscle relaxants, abdominal or chest surgery, pneumonia, *asthma*, liver or kidney disorders, trauma, a *stroke* or a brain tumour involving the breathing centre in the brain.

WHAT YOU CAN DO

Many hiccup remedies use a voluntary breathing technique in order to interrupt the involuntary spasm of the diaphragm. Others divert your attention from the hiccups to reduce the *anxiety* or tension helping to cause them.

- Take a deep breath and hold for a count of 30.

- Drink cold water from the opposite side of a glass.

- Crunch some crushed ice.

- Chew something with a powerful flavour – and really concentrate on the taste. Ginger is good because it also relieves *indigestion*. Other suitable nibbles include raw garlic, ripe stilton cheese, a spice clove, a strong peppermint or an aniseed ball.

- Aniseed is a traditional hiccup remedy. For a troublesome attack which won't quite go away, pound some aniseeds using a pestle and mortar or place between two layers of paper and hammer them hard to release their oil. Steep in boiling water for 10 minutes, strain and sip slowly.

Two diversionary techniques
- Bring your hands in front of you at waist level. Interlock your fingers tightly and pull hard as though trying to separate them. Take a deep breath and pull to a count of 20–30.

- Stand on one leg, with your eyes closed if possible. You can hold your arms out to the sides to help you balance, but don't touch a wall or furniture.

> **CAUTION:** Do not attempt this if you have had too much to drink or suffer from any disability which may cause you to fall.

- *Acupressure* – work on Abdominal Sorrow.
- *Relaxation* or hypnotherapy may help where tension and stress are a problem.
- Practise regular *Yoga.*

Drug remedies

○ There is no specific medication for persistent or powerful hiccups in common use, but various treatments have been attempted, including eating dry sugar (which you also try as a home remedy).

> ### SEE YOUR DOCTOR IF...
>
> - Your hiccup attacks are frequent or fail to improve with self-treatment.
> - Surgery to the phrenic nerve interrupts the stimuli producing hiccups. This would only be considered in rare cases.

■ Hoarseness and Loss of Voice

Hoarseness is often due to laryngitis (inflammation of the larynx or voice box). When laryngitis is acute and short-lived, you become hoarse for a day or so and may lose your voice later if the infection persists. Such attacks are generally due to a *cold, flu* or throat virus, although your throat may not actually become sore, and you tend to sound worse than you feel.

Chronic laryngitis can result from the passive and active smoking, inhaling noxious fumes, drinking too much or prolonged vomiting and can be an occupational hazard in certain jobs.

WHAT YOU CAN DO

- Keep away from polluted atmospheres and stop smoking.

- Treat a *sore throat, cold* or *flu* as recommended.

- Drink plenty of fluids, including freshly squeezed vegetable and fruit juices. Apple, lettuce and celery have a calming effect. Carrot, beetroot and cucumber help to boost resistance.

- Sip warm lemon balm or chamomile tea to soothe a tired throat and help you relax.

- *Rest your voice* – regardless of the cause of your laryngitis, do not strain to talk, shout or sing. Over-reaching the voice is an occupational hazard for singers, actors learning to project their voices and teachers, parents, prison officers and drilling sergeants, all of whom are prone to a great deal of shouting daily.

- Steam inhalations relieve laryngeal inflammation and spasm, reducing the swelling and distortion of the vocal cords. Adding a few drops of essential oil of benzoin, borneol, eucalyptus, hyssop, myrrh, pine, sage, sandalwood or tea tree enhances the benefits of the steam and helps to kill the germs.

- Use these homoeopathic remedies for an acute attack especially where infection is present (take four times daily for up to seven days):

  - For symptoms that start suddenly and are aggravated by cold dry winds, with fever and restlessness: Aconite 30c

  - For loss of voice and a dry barking *cough*: Spongia 6c

  - For a throat that feels worse in the morning and in cold dry winds, feels better indoors in the warm, has a *choking* sensation and loose *cough* producing yellow phlegm: Hepar sulph. 6c

  - For an elderly person whose throat is worse in the evening and in cold damp weather, has poor circulation and feels cold but breaks out in sweats: Carbo veg. 6c

- Specific remedies for singers, to be taken four times daily for up to three days:

  - For a voice feeble from overuse and a tickle in larynx worsened by the cold: Alumina 6c

  - For increased tickle and a voice that is weak, trembly and inclined to break: Argentum 6c

  - For a voice weak on starting to sing but improved after a few minutes: Rhus tox. 6c

  - For a clear discharge from the nose, tender larynx, hurts to sing: Phosphorus 6c

Drug remedies

- Use *cold* and/or *sore throat* remedies as needed.

- Karvol capsules and similar products which release eucalyptus, menthol, pine, etc. when dissolved in hot water and inhaled in steam.

SEE YOUR DOCTOR IF...

- Simple remedies fail to relieve the hoarseness.
- You have been emotionally strained – non-infective laryngitis can be caused by stress, anxiety and worry.

■ Nosebleeds

Bleeding from the nose, known as epistaxis, is usually caused by a punch or fall, a trivial blow or jolt. The flexible lower end of your nose below the bony 'bridge' is the usual source of bleeding, particularly the vessels within the tip, just below the lining. These veins bleed readily if damaged or inflamed by heavy *colds*, for example, or *hayfever*.

Causes other than injury and inflammation include *high blood pressure*, childhood fevers, mountain sickness and air flight cabin depressurization. Nasal polyps – harmless swellings in the nasal lining – also make nosebleeds more likely.

You may have felt alarmed at the amount of blood a nosebleed can produce, but the correct first aid procedures quickly stem the flow. Nosebleeds need prompt and effective treatment, but they are not dangerous unless you are on anticoagulants to prevent clotting, for example warfarin, or suffer from a blood clotting disorder like haemophilia.

WHAT YOU CAN DO

- If an attack starts, sit down and lean forward to let blood drain from nose. Breathe through mouth and pinch soft part of nose.

CAUTION: send to hospital if nose bleed is severe and lasts for longer than 30 minutes.

- If you are prone to nosebleeds, avoid rough and tumble games in which your face is a likely target.
- Wear a nose shield for any contact sports.
- Take remedies promptly for *colds*, catarrh, *hayfever*, etc., to reduce sneezing attacks, nasal inflammation and frequent wiping.
- Avoid long-term use of steroid sprays for nasal congestion – they thin the skin and increase the risks of bleeds. (SEE *other treatments for nasal congestion* in *Colds* and *Hayfever*.)
- Blow your nose as gently as you can.
- Avoid very dry atmospheres where possible, or use a humidifier.
- Combat stress with regular *relaxation* and/or *Yoga*.
- Try these homoeopathic remedies every 2 minutes for up to 10 doses:
  - Nosebleed follows an injury: Arnica 6c
  - Where blood is bright red: Ipecac 6c
  - Bleed brought on by violent nose-blowing: Phosphorus 6c
  - Nosebleed with a headache which is worsened by leaning forwards: Hamamelis – 6c
  - Bright red blood, person feels faint, especially if they look rather pale: Ferrum phos. 6c
  - In all other cases: Vipera 6c
- Try *acupressure* on these points:
  - Eyes Bright
  - Facial Beauty
  - Joining the Valley – if nosebleeds are frequent and unexplained.

> **CAUTION:** Avoid if pregnant until labour because the use of this point can cause premature contractions.

  - Middle of a Person

Drug remedies

○ Mouthwashes, gargles and throat sprays may prove helpful.

SEE YOUR DOCTOR IF...

- Your nose is always stuffy, but you don't have a *cold* or *hayfever* – they will examine you for nasal polyps and refer you to an ENT (ear, nose and throat) specialist if required.
- You are on anti-coagulant therapy and nosebleeds have just started – your INR (reflection of the blood's thinness) needs checking urgently.
- If you are not on anti-coagulants, but you're getting nosebleeds and other related symptoms like tiredness, *mouth ulcers* or unexplained *bruising*. You need a full examination and blood tests.

▪ Sinusitis

This is inflammation of the sinuses, air spaces inside the bones of the face. Sinusitis can occur alone, but often accompanies *hayfever* or a *cold*. Inflammation inside the nose spreads into the sinuses via a small opening through which their fluid normally drains. If this opening becomes blocked, pressure builds up within the sinuses and the trapped fluid becomes infected. You feel pain due to the inflamed membranes lining the sinuses and the pressure of the infected mucus within them. You may develop a runny or blocked nose, a fever and a painful, tender forehead, cheekbones, upper jaw and teeth.

Mild sinusitis accompanying a head *cold* usually settles within a few days, but you will need a course of antibiotics if a high fever and severe pain suggest a bacterial infection.

WHAT YOU CAN DO

- Eat healthily to strengthen your immune system. Avoid animal fats and dairy products because they stimulate mucus production.

- Avoid smoking and smoky atmospheres.

- Towel-over-head steam inhalations can loosen mucus, reduce inflammation and help to unblock sinuses. Essential oil of benzoin, cajeput, eucalyptus, niaouli or tea tree are all helpful. After inhaling, add 3 drops of any of these to 10 mls (2 tsp) carrier oil, and rub gently into the outside of your nose and over tender facial areas.

- An air ionizer can be very helpful when your nose is congested.

- To shift thick catarrh, simmer one to two slices of fresh ginger root in a mug of water for 10 minutes. Add a couple of fresh (or pinch of dried) sage leaves (which also combat mucus), a pinch of cinnamon for flavour and a teaspoonful of honey for its antibiotic action. Sip and savour it.

- Take some Siberian ginseng to help overcome the infection.

- *Acupressure* can be beneficial. Try:

  ○ Heavenly Pillar – I discovered the benefits of this area by accident when massaging the back of my neck to relieve a *headache.* Suddenly my sinuses cleared (as well as the *headache*), and I could breathe more freely than I had for months!

  ○ Welcoming Perfume

- The *Yoga* asanas Corpse and Shoulder Stand are recommended for sinusitis.

Drug remedies

o Aspirin, paracetamol or ibuprofen to reduce fever and ease the pain.

o Alternatively, a stronger painkiller such as a paracetamol + codeine combination.

o Steam inhalation, for example of Friar's balsam.

o Decongestant nasal drops or tablets can help.

o Antibiotics when a bacterial infection is present.

SEE YOUR DOCTOR IF...

• You have a persistent fever and/or pain despite home remedies.
• You regularly suffer sinusitis attacks – a small operation may help. Often carried out under local anaesthetic, this aims to enlarge the opening in the nasal cavity, wash out the infected sinuses and enable their secretions to drain more easily.

■ Snoring and Sleep Apnoea

When you are asleep, your throat muscles relax and sag. Excessive sagging obstructs your air supply, which has to be forced through a narrow gap down into your lungs. Your soft upper palate on the roof of your mouth and your uvula, the dangly fleshy bit between your tonsils, then vibrate extra-rapidly, producing snores. Sleeping on your back worsens the problem, because your tongue falls back, forcing the uvula against the back of your throat.

In sleep apnoea (Greek, meaning 'breathlessness'), you stop breathing for repeated cycles of 10–30 seconds, which reduces your brain's oxygen supply. You may snort loudly and wake abruptly, gasping for breath and with jerking limbs. And as your system is on constant alert to wake you if your breathing becomes obstructed, you are likely to suffer from chronic tiredness.

Triggers for over-relaxed throat muscles include a blocked nose, *sinusitis, hayfever,* allergies to wheat, eggs and house dust mites, big tonsils, a deformed upper airway or uvula, obesity, smoking, excessive alcohol intake, sleeping pills and *cough* mixtures containing dextromethorphan. Snoring also tends to run in families.

WHAT YOU CAN DO

- Add a pillow to elevate your head or raise the head of your bed by 10 cms (4 inches).

- Shed excess weight.

- Avoid sleeping pills and replace an alcoholic nightcap with a warm milky drink.

- Avoid heavy meals and rich high-fat foods before bedtime. An overtaxed digestive system diverts blood from the brain, aggravating the effects of oxygen shortage, while a loaded stomach presses upwards on the diaphragm, impeding breathing.

- Stop smoking. Cigarettes, especially before bedtime, can irritate the throat lining, causing it to swell.

- Towel-over-head steam inhalations help to open your airway – choose from bergamot, cajeput and chamomile essential oils.

- Various devices can help to keep the nostrils widely dilated when you sleep. You can achieve a similar effect with two Band-Aids running from the nose to each cheek.

- Try natural anti-snoring sprays. SnoreStop Extinguisher and YSNORE Antisnore Nasal Spray contain safe effective homoeopathic remedies. Both are advertised on the internet and your pharmacist can recommend others.

Drug remedies

- Antiseptic mouthwashes will help to clear any excess mucus (SEE *Sore Throat*).

- A steroidal nasal spray combats nasal stuffiness and may help to reduce mouth breathing.

SEE YOUR DOCTOR IF...

- You suffer from sleep apnoea, a potentially serious condition linked to increased risks of *high blood pressure*, heart disease and *strokes*. Clinical studies have confirmed raised blood levels of the amino acid homocysteine in sufferers, probably due to free radical damage. Free radicals attack blood vessel linings, encouraging clogging and LDLs (low density lipoproteins), which help to counteract harmful HDL cholesterol. Recent studies have also suggested sleep apnoea's role in triggering type II diabetes. Raised carbon dioxide levels trigger high levels of the stress hormones adrenaline and noradrenaline, interfering with insulin's control of blood sugar levels (SEE *Blood Sugar Imbalance*). Your doctor may refer you to a sleep laboratory to investigate your sleep apnoea. Surgery can sometimes correct severe snoring and sleep apnoea.

▪ Sore Throat and Tonsillitis

The first symptom of a sore throat could be a dry throat, followed by painful swallowing. Occasionally a smoky atmosphere, talking too much or shouting may be responsible, but if an infection is present, you develop other symptoms too. Your throat looks red and raw, and inflamed tonsils appear as bright crimson lumps like cherry tomatoes at the back of your throat, coated with whitish-yellow pus if the infection is bacterial. The lymph glands in your neck become tender and swollen, and you may also develop muscular aches, a *headache, difficulty in swallowing* liquids and solids, a runny nose and fever (SEE *The Common Cold, Hayfever*).

Most throat infections are caused by viruses and are easy to treat with home remedies, but a severe sore throat or tonsillitis is frequently due to bacteria, for which antibiotics are needed. Children up to the age of 12 with tonsillitis tend to develop tummyache rather than a sore throat and they usually refuse to eat or drink and vomit. This is because lymph glands in the abdomen become inflamed and tender and gastric symptoms take precedence over the throat problem.

WHAT YOU CAN DO

- Viral and bacterial throat infections are passed on by inhaling infected droplets, so wherever possible steer clear of sufferers' *coughs* and *colds*.

- Drink at least eight glasses of water daily plus extra-fresh juice to avoid a parched throat. Combat smoky, stuffy, dry atmospheres with fresh air, outdoor exercise and a humidifier (use a purpose-made machine or stand bowls of water around rooms with radiators).

- Avoid obvious sources of infection such as sucking a baby's dummy straight after the baby has sucked it or after it has been spat out or dropped on the floor. Don't swap or reuse cups, glasses and cutlery without washing them, and don't let pets lick you on or around your mouth or eat off your plate.

- Give up smoking and persuade family members to do so too.

- Consider buying an air ionizer.

- Help prevent sore throats by gargling night and morning with a glass of water with one added drop of essential oil of benzoin, cajeput, eucalyptus, rosemary or tea tree. If a sore throat develops, gargle four to five times daily with a glass of water containing 2½ ml (½ tsp) of salt or two added drops of any of the above essences or of cinnamon, clove, ginger or hyssop.

- To clear mucus, sip iced water mixed with fresh pineapple juice. If you crave a warming drink, sip hot lemon and honey, spiced up with grated ginger root or flavoured with congestion-beating mint or sage.

- Suck an antiseptic, herbal, zinc or propolis throat lozenge (propolis is a natural antibacterial substance which bees make to keep their hives infection-free).

- Calendula herbal remedies are often recommended for tonsillitis and swollen glands.

Drug remedies

○ Antiseptic gargles and mouthwashes.

○ Paracetamol or ibuprofen.

○ Throat pastilles.

SEE YOUR DOCTOR IF...

- You or your child has tonsillitis.
- Your sore throat worsens despite home measures and/or antibiotics.
- You are having increasing *difficulty in swallowing* or problems swallowing liquids.
- You develop a high fever and feel very unwell.

10

Heart and Blood Vessel Ailments

• Angina • Deep vein thrombosis (DVT) • Fainting attacks • High blood pressure • Palpitations • Poor circulation in the feet • Poor circulation in the hands • Restless legs • Stroke • Varicose veins

---

■ Angina

Angina is pain in heart muscle deprived of oxygen. This happens when the coronary arteries supplying the heart become clogged with fatty deposits, reducing the volume of blood they can deliver. When the heart has to beat more quickly, there is too little blood – and therefore oxygen – to meet its needs. Waste products such as lactic acid accumulate, causing pain in the heart's muscular walls.

You will have experienced something similar if you have over-taxed your calf muscles by a steep walk or climb. Your arteries and circulation, unused to the demand, will have carried too little blood to your leg muscles, and waste products will have gathered, causing pain.

Angina symptoms include pain or a tight clamping sensation in the middle/left chest, extending and down one or both arms and/or up into the jaw. You may also feel sick, hot and faint. Angina triggers include exercise and strong emotion such as intense excitement, fear, rage or shock.

WHAT YOU CAN DO

- You can help to prevent angina by a healthy diet, regular exercise and losing surplus weight.

- Stop smoking, reduce your alcohol intake, have regular blood pressure and cholesterol checks and learn to relax.

- A low intake of total and animal-derived fat, sodium-based salt, sugar and other refined carbohydrates is axiomatic to improved heart health. Five daily portions of fresh fruit and vegetables provide antioxidants which help to prevent dangerous LDL cholesterol from clogging arteries.

- Aubergines, garlic, onions, apples, pectin (found in apples and the white membranes of citrus fruit), soya beans and yoghurt all help to lower cholesterol.

- Magnesium helps the heart maintain a normal rhythm. You will find it in fish and seafood, nuts, soya products, green leafy vegetables and sunflower seeds, which also curb nicotine cravings.

- Yeast and torula yeast contain co-enzyme Q10, a vitamin-like nutrient which specifically enhances oxygen utilization in heart cells (it is also available as a supplement).

- Fresh undiluted beetroot juice is said to dissolve calcium deposits (sometimes found in arterial walls) and to relieve raised blood pressure and coronary artery disorders. Drink 300 ml (½ pint) daily mixed with the same quantity of carrot juice.

- Take regular exercise that challenges and strengthens the heart and lungs. A qualified fitness instructor can work out a suitable regimen, working with your GP or specialist if you are extremely overweight and/or already suffer from angina.

- Prioritize learning to relax. *Yoga*, t'ai chi and *relaxation* are hugely beneficial to angina sufferers.

- See a hypnotherapist or counsellor to help you cope with negative emotions.

- Useful *Bach Flower Remedies* include Red Chestnut, to help restore trust, and Holly to help you cope with anger, desire for revenge, suspicions and jealousy.

Drug remedies

o Short-acting glyceryl trinitrate, available as a spray and tablets to chew or dissolve on or below the tongue, is usually used to relieve angina attacks in progress.

o Sustained-release glyceryl trinitrate and isosorbide (also a nitrate) are used to help prevent attacks.

SEE YOUR DOCTOR IF...

- You experience unexplained chest pain.
- Prescribed medicines are not working.
- Home remedies fail to help.

■ Deep Vein Thrombosis

You are probably aware of the dangers of deep vein thrombosis from its intensive media coverage. Most of us associate DVT with long-haul flights, but any cramped seating that confines your movements for hours can be responsible. It's dangerous because a clot or thrombus formed in a deep leg vein (SEE *Varicose Veins*) not only obstructs the passage of blood back to the pelvis but can also break up, releasing fragments (emboli) into the bloodstream. Pulmonary embolism, where a clot reaches the lungs, can prove fatal.

With DVT, you would notice a pain deep within your calf muscle or lower abdomen, with swelling and tightness of the affected area. The skin over a thrombus would become inflamed and movement would be painful, especially bending your toes upwards towards your face when lying down with your legs stretched out straight. Doctors use this technique, called Homan's test, when a patient has DVT symptoms. A sudden stab of pain in the calf strongly suggests a positive diagnosis.

WHAT YOU CAN DO

- Avoid cramped, confined seating wherever possible. When driving, get out, walk about and stretch every hour or so. When an air passenger, walk to the lavatory as often as you can and stretch your leg muscles regularly. Follow the leg exercise routines suggested by flight attendants or others and wear flight support socks/stockings, especially on long-haul flights.

- Avoid constricting clothing and seat or safety belts – adjust the latter to suit your size and shape.

- Avoid oral contraceptives and hormone replacement therapy (HRT) if you or close relatives have ever suffered from thrombosis.

- Make sure you drink six to eight glasses of water daily and drink extra water when travelling. For 24 hours prior to flying and on the flight itself, avoid alcohol and rich fatty foods, and drink freshly squeezed juices. Try this pre-flight recipe: To 250 ml

(½ pint) of carrot juice, add celery, which combats fluid retention and swelling, lettuce, for its calming effects, and a little watercress or spinach to purify the blood. Sip twice daily and take some in a flask for the flight.

- Follow a wholefood diet, including citrus fruit and other sources of vitamin C with bioflavonoids (which improve sluggish circulation in the legs) and wheatgerm, egg yolks, wholegrain cereals and green leafy vegetables to supply vitamin E (which helps to prevent and dissolve blood clots).

- Medical herbalists might prescribe preparations of butcher's broom or gotu kola to improve the circulation and combat clotting. Tonka (or Tonquin) beans contain an anti-coagulant similar to the body's own. Use under professional supervision. Extract of Irish moss (carragheen), the vegetarian equivalent of gelatine, helps to reduce the risks of all types of thrombosis.

- Use the same *aromatherapy* leg massage oil recommended for *restless legs* to cut the risks of – *but not to treat* – DVT.

- Try these homoeopathic remedies 2 hourly for up to 6 doses while awaiting diagnosis and treatment for DVT:

  - For symptoms on the left-hand side, with pain and swelling and *poor circulation in feet and hands*: Lachesis 6c

  - For right-sided symptoms, cold swollen limbs and *bruising*: Bothrops 6c

  - For DVT with severe pain, exhaustion and *varicose veins*: Hamamelis 6c

Drug remedies

- Anti-coagulant drugs to prevent clotting, selected according to the patient's unique requirements.

- Clot-dispersing drugs if needed.

SEE YOUR DOCTOR IF...

- You experience symptoms suggestive of DVT.
- You have any unexplained calf or thigh swelling, pain or inflammation.

■ Fainting Attacks

Fainting attacks are due to insufficient blood, and therefore oxygen, reaching the brain: falling lowers the head, restoring the blood supply and consciousness. Symptoms include objects 'swimming' around you, black dots before your eyes and feeling hot, sweaty and possibly nauseous. You slump or fall to the ground and come to moments or minutes later. Your body may jerk in a seizure-like way while you are 'out', due to oxygen shortage to the brain.

Physical causes include standing still long enough for your blood to pool in your legs and getting up too quickly after a rest for your blood vessels to readjust in time. Powerful emotion can also be responsible. It stimulates the release of adrenaline and noradrenaline preparing you for 'fight or flight'. Blood is diverted to your main muscle groups and your heart pumps more slowly, temporarily depriving your brain.

Fortunately, fainting is less common now than in past centuries, when women fainted – or had 'the vapours' – much more frequently. We are all more used to unpleasant sights and emotional trauma nowadays, and we're free of the tight bodices which used to restrict blood flow to the upper parts of the body.

WHAT YOU CAN DO

- When standing still for long periods, squeeze and relax your calf and thighs muscles regularly or shift your weight from one foot to the other to encourage the flow of blood upwards.

- Get up slowly after lying or sitting. Some heart and blood pressure drugs increase the risks of blacking out when you get up, due to a momentary drop in blood pressure ('postural hypotension').

- Avoid hot stuffy atmospheres and wear loosely fitting clothes, especially around your waist and neck.

- If you feel faint, sit or lie down so that your head is lower than your body. Try to get some fresh air and splash your face and neck with cold water. (SEE ALSO *First Aid*.)

- A wholefood diet (SEE *Nutritional Medicine*) supplies anti-oxidants and other nutrients vital to a healthy heart and blood vessels. Anaemia increases the risks of fainting, so ensure that you are getting adequate iron in your diet, and ask your doctor for a blood test if you have heavy periods (SEE *Heavy Vaginal Bleeding*) or are breastfeeding.

- Lavender water, smelling salts and Eau de Cologne work as well for fainting attacks today as they did in the past. Lavender-scented ammonium crystals rapidly restore consciousness if held to the nose. You can also dab the cologne or lavender essential oil onto your temples, or add a few drops (or of lemon, mandarin, orange or petitgrain oil) to cold water to bathe your face or make up a forehead compress.

- Homoeopathic remedies to take every 5 minutes for up to 7 doses when faintness threatens or on regaining full consciousness:

  - For symptoms-triggered fainting, with a weak and trembly feeling: Gelsemium 6c

  - For fainting at sight of blood: Nux 6c

○ For fainting after emotional shock: Ignatia 6c

○ For fainting triggered by fright, when you are numb with shock: Opium 6c

Drug remedies

○ There are no specific medicines for fainting attacks. Smelling salts and 4711 Eau de Cologne are available from some pharmacies.

SEE YOUR DOCTOR IF...

- You frequently faint.
- You think you may be anaemic.
- Your blood pressure medication makes you feel dizzy or faint.

▪ High Blood Pressure

High blood pressure – hypertension – is sometimes called the 'silent killer' because it produces so few symptoms. Many sufferers, however, know when their blood pressure climbs. Possible symptoms include feeling light-headed, slightly dizzy or 'not quite with it' and/or a particular kind of *headache*, especially on waking.

'Normal' blood pressure is approximately 120/80 mm mercury; the first, or systolic, pressure represents the heart's pumping force, and the second, or diastolic, pressure the resistance put up by the arterial circulation. Blood pressure varies as you exercise, rest, become stressed, etc., and it does rise slightly with age. But because hypertension damages the heart, blood vessels, kidneys and other organs and is a major risk factor for heart attacks and *strokes*, doctors aim to achieve readings below 140/85, depending upon the patient's age and other health factors.

Eighty per cent of all hypertension arises for no discernible reason, but the remaining 20 per cent is caused by diseased arteries, kidneys or (occasionally) adrenal glands.

WHAT YOU CAN DO

- Have regular BP checks and take medication as prescribed (SEE *page 167*).

- Keep your weight within normal limits for your height and build.

- Stop smoking and keep to the guidelines for safe drinking.

- Eat low-salt, low-saturated-fat wholefoods, including five daily portions of fresh fruit and vegetables. Their antioxidants help to keep arteries healthy and combat clot formation.

- Use cold-pressed olive or other unprocessed vegetable oil for cooking, salad dressings, etc.

- Drink some raw fruit or vegetable juice daily. Try 300–600 ml (½–1 pint) of one or more of the following: celery, cucumber, grapefruit, orange, pear or pineapple. Stir in 5 ml (1 tsp) runny honey to calm your nerves, or add the honey to 20 ml (4 tsp) cider vinegar and sip slowly, savouring the flavour (this also makes a pleasant salad dressing, mixed with chopped herbs).

- Recommended supplements (doses according to directions) include evening primrose oil, co-enzyme Q10, pollen, lecithin, vitamin E, selenium, magnesium, garlic, fish oil (or eat garlic raw plus three to four portions oily fish weekly, for example mackerel, sardines, tuna).

- Most importantly, learn *relaxation* techniques which you can practise under stress. *Yoga*, t'ai chi, deep *relaxation* and meditation are extremely beneficial.

- Hypnotherapy can teach you various techniques to calm body and mind.

- Calm yourself with chamomile or lime-flower tea, and have baths perfumed with soothing ylang ylang, which helps to regulate the heart rate.

- *Bach Flower Remedies* relevant to *palpitations* and *angina* may be suitable for high blood pressure sufferers.

Drug remedies

○ Diuretics (water pills), for example bendroflumethiazide.

○ Beta blockers, for example propranolol, atenolol.

○ Calcium antagonists, which regulate muscle tone in the heart and circulation, for example diltiazem, nifedipine.

Angiotensin-converting enzyme (ACE) inhibitors which help to prevent arterial spasm, for example perindopril, captopril.

SEE YOUR DOCTOR IF...

- You are taking the contraceptive pill or are being treated for hypertension. You need a BP check every 6 months (once yearly if you are fit).
- Your blood pressure medication does not suit you – there's always an alternative.
- You need advice and help to lose weight.

- You have chest *pains*, blackouts, *headaches*, falls, *dizzy spells* or other unexplained symptoms.
- Simple remedies fail to help.

■ Palpitations

You do not usually notice your heart beating, but if you suffer from palpitations you may experience a flutter inside your chest or feel your heart racing, thudding, beating unevenly or apparently threatening to stop. Palpitations usually come on at rest, without any of the triggers such as a fright, exercise or excitement that set the normal heart pounding.

If your heart is healthy, palpitations are nothing to worry about – you may feel nauseous or faint, but this can result as much from fear as from a heart problem. Investigations often fail to identify a cause, but common triggers include nicotine, caffeine, alcohol, *anxiety* and panic attacks, low blood sugar (hypoglycaemia) (SEE *Blood Sugar Imbalance*) and an overactive thyroid gland.

A defect within the heart's pacemaker, the sino-atrial (SA) node, is occasionally to blame. You may need medication, a small operation or, occasionally, a pacemaker to restore normal rhythm.

WHAT YOU CAN DO

- Eliminate spicy dishes, alcohol, stuffy atmospheres, strong tea, coffee and colas, and very hot showers and baths.

- Stop smoking.

- Learn to relax – it is usually as beneficial as any prescription medicine. Relieve anger, anxiety and frustration with regular exercise, and try deep *relaxation, Yoga,* t'ai chi, Pilates or some other activity that stretches and relaxes knotted muscles while teaching breath control. (Check first with your doctor.)

- Hypnotherapy can teach therapeutic visualization and *relaxation* of mind and body.

- To cope with a racing pulse, sit or stand quietly and take slow deep breaths. Say 'R-E-L-A-X' as you exhale, picturing your heart beating more calmly and slowly.

- Find the pulse in your neck on *one side only*. Gentle, firm pressure maintained for 30–40 seconds, till the pulse disappears, slows a racing heart.

- Eat healthy wholefoods with plenty of calming juices (in addition to six to eight glasses of water daily). Freshly squeezed carrot, celery and apple juice and carrot, lettuce and cucumber are great nerve-soothers. Fresh fruit and vegetables rich in antioxidants may help reduce attacks – globe artichokes, in particular, are often recommended for this purpose.

- Calming herbal teas include basil, chamomile, lime flower, orange leaf and rose petal. You can make your own version with a mixture of the fresh ingredients.

- Liquorice and liquorice water (made by dissolving sticks of the natural solidified juice) are also beneficial.

- Cider vinegar on a sugar lump or mixed with a little runny honey or added to a tumbler of water is said to stop palpitations.

- Homoeopathic remedies – take every 5 minutes for up to 6 doses:

  ○ For palpitations triggered by too much to eat or drink, or after expending nervous energy when feeling cold and grumpy: Nux 6c

  ○ For palpitations with faintness, *anxiety*, tightness in chest, especially when linked to the menopause: Lachesis 6c

- Combine any of the above with a *Bach Flower Remedy*. Red Chestnut helps persistent *anxiety*, Aspen helps trembling apprehension and haunting fears, White Chestnut reduces circling thoughts and mental turmoil.

Drug remedies

○ Propranolol, a beta blocker drug (SEE *High Blood Pressure*) can slow a racing heart caused by *anxiety*.

○ Verapamil is one of many drugs prescribed for abnormal heart rhythms.

SEE YOUR DOCTOR IF...

- You have a recurrent problem with your pulse or heart beat.
- You experience additional symptoms such as *fainting attacks, heavy perspiration, dizzy spells* and chest pain.
- Simple home measures are ineffective.

▪ Poor Circulation in the Feet

If your leg arteries are clogged, blood circulation to your feet is reduced. Your toes, feet and lower legs probably look white and feel chilly in bed and in cold weather, however warm your socks.

If the furring up is severe, walking may be painful. Reduced blood, oxygen and nutrients reach your lower limb muscles, and waste metabolic products, for example lactic acid, accumulate, triggering pain. You are forced to rest after a certain distance. This will steadily decrease as your arteries become more blocked. Sufferers typically limp with pain if they try to drive themselves on once the pain has started. You may eventually suffer pain at rest and the tissues of your feet and toes could become gangrenous without prompt medical treatment or surgery.

This condition, claudication, is named after the Roman emperor Claudius, who walked with a halting gait (although not necessarily as a result of arterial disease).

WHAT YOU CAN DO

- Lose surplus weight and give up smoking.

- Exercise regularly, choosing routines that work all your main muscle groups, especially those of the legs. If you already suffer from claudication or arterial blockage, follow exercise routines as recommended and walk as far as you are advised daily.

- Follow the diet recommended for *angina*. Foods rich in anti-oxidants beta-carotene (vitamin A), vitamin B complex, vitamin C and bioflavonoids, vitamin E, zinc, calcium, magnesium and selenium are especially beneficial (SEE *Nutritional Medicine*).

- The naturally occurring calcium + magnesium supplement dolomite helps to relieve calf cramps, including those that occur in the night due to poor circulation. Vitamin E supplements are reputed to do the same. Try either or both for a month or so, or seek expert advice from a nutritionist who will monitor your intake of these nutrients from dietary or supplementary sources.

- Juice some freshly scrubbed carrots together with a head of broccoli florets or three handfuls of spinach leaves to top up your vitamin and mineral levels.

- Add a few drops of cypress, lavender or lemon oil to a warm (not hot) bath or to a self-massaging footbath to improve the circulation in your feet.

- You can also massage some wintergreen cream into your feet and calves to improve the local circulation, as it boosts blood flow (avoid any scratches or broken skin).

- The herb valerian is best known for its sleep-inducing properties, but it also relaxes blood vessel spasm and may be recommended as part of a treatment programme for mild small artery disease.

- Red clover relieves smooth muscle spasm in the arterioles (smallest arteries) of the legs. Its powerful antioxidant properties also promote tissue repair and may help to protect affected blood vessels from further damage.

Drug remedies

○ Drugs which dilate blood vessels and improve circulation.

○ Nicotinic acid derivatives such as inositol nicotinate, taken as tablets.

○ Cilostazol (in tablet form) which combats clot formation and extends pain-free walking distance when there is no pain at rest or peripheral tissue damage.

○ Cinnarizine (capsules), an antihistamine with blood vessel dilating properties.

SEE YOUR DOCTOR IF...

- You experience lower limb pain on walking – you need medical attention.
- Simple remedies to promote healthy blood flow do not work.

▪ Poor Circulation in the Hands

If you suffer from poor circulation in the hands then you will know how hard everyday tasks become in cold weather. Writing, counting change, doing up poppers and zips, using keys, etc. can all present problems.

Cold temperatures make skin vessels contract, diverting blood to deeper tissues in an attempt to conserve body heat. But in the condition known as Raynaud's phenomenon (RP), small arteries in the hands (and occasionally feet) contract at normal temperatures, one or more fingers go white and numb, and pins and needles sometimes develop when the blood flow returns to normal. Triggers include continued vibration (for example in pneumatic drill workers), beta blockers and other drugs, stress and negative emotion, and the cold and damp.

Chilblains develop when surface blood vessels contract, depriving the skin of blood and oxygen. They appear as small inflamed and intensely itchy swellings on fingers, toes, ears or nose, sometimes with broken skin which weeps and can become infected.

WHAT YOU CAN DO

- Wrap up warmly and wear inner and outer gloves in cold damp weather.

- If you have RP, immerse your hand or affected fingers in warm water and massage the fingers from the base to the tips.

- Treat chilblains promptly to avoid open sores. Avoid handling snow or ice (unless obliged to, and then with gloves), and dry hands well after immersion in water.

- Don't scratch chilblains – this tears the skin.

- A wholefood diet with five or more daily helpings of fresh raw fruit or vegetables (and their juices) supplies antioxidants for healthy blood vessels. Protein from fish, poultry, lean meat, low-fat dairy, pulses, grains and nuts provides amino acids for repairing and replacing worn-out tissues.

- A reduced fat intake with most dietary fats coming from unprocessed vegetable oils reduces the risks of fat-clogged arteries. Polyunsaturated fatty acids found in cold-pressed olive, sunflower and safflower oil and oily fish are also beneficial.

- Antioxidant bioflavonoids found naturally with vitamin C are clinically proven to strengthen small blood vessels. They are found in the white pith and membranes of citrus fruit and also in apricots, blackberries, buckwheat, cherries and rosehips. Try sachets of rosehip tea, flavouring if needed with a little honey.

- For RP or chilblains, holistic therapists may recommend hand baths, tepid at first and gradually becoming warmer, to relieve the acute symptoms. Add a handful of fresh or dried elderflowers to enhance blood flow. Regular hand baths of warm alternating with cool water can stimulate and help to 're-educate' the circulation.

- Massage the upper trunk, shoulders and arms to improve blood flow to the hands with 10 mls (2 tbsp) almond oil mixed with two to three drops of essence of bryony, lemon or lavender once or twice daily.

- Dab chilblains with freshly cut onion or garlic, or tea tree oil. Apply calendula cream with or without St John's wort extract if the skin is broken.

- Take the homoeopathic remedy Agaricus 6c half hourly for up to six doses for burning, itching, swollen chilblains unrelieved by cool temperatures, and apply Tamus ointment.

Drug remedies

○ Moxisylyte (an alpha-blocker) is prescribed for short-term control of RP.

○ Cinnarizine for more advanced RP.

○ For chilblains, use Savlon antiseptic cream or Balmosa rubifacient containing (among others) menthol, camphor and an aspirin compound.

SEE YOUR DOCTOR IF...

• Simple home treatments do not help.

■ Restless Legs

If you're a poor sleeper, restless legs may be to blame. Affecting 5–10 per cent of adults, this is a major cause of *insomnia*, although studies have shown that many sufferers complain of disturbed nights rather than their legs, attributing their restlessness to a sleeping problem.

Alternatively, you may be only too aware of tingling, prickling, burning feelings in your lower legs that come on at rest and are worse at night. Unable to keep still and with your legs sometimes jerking involuntarily, you gain relief only in constant leg movement and/or in getting out of bed and walking about. Like *snoring*, your restless legs can become a problem for your partner, whose slumber may frequently be disturbed by inadvertent kicks and your continually changing position.

The most important causes are a minor problem with the brain neurones controlling voluntary movement and the inefficient drainage of blood from the lower limbs (SEE *Varicose Veins*). Other triggers include caffeine, withdrawal from alcohol or tranquillizer dependence, diabetes and a lack of iron or vitamin B.

WHAT YOU CAN DO

- Eat healthily and encourage blood to drain away from your legs as advised for *varicose veins*.

- Make sure of an adequate iron supply from lean red meat and offal, egg yolks, wheatgerm, cheddar cheese, seaweed, nuts and lentils. Obtain vitamin B from wholewheat flour and its products, beef, kidney and liver, sunflower seeds and cashew nuts, and bioflavonoids from citrus fruit, paw paw, grapes, tomatoes, green peppers, broccoli and cherries. Folic acid and vitamin E are also important.

- Cool compresses soothe the burning sensation even when the skin feels cool to the touch. Add some witch hazel tincture or solution to a compress, or dab on fiery leg areas according to the packet instructions.

- Medical herbalists may prescribe preparations of butcher's broom to be taken an hour before bed. Chamomile tea is a mild sedative and can also relieve muscular spasms.

- Give your legs a regular *aromatherapy* massage. To 15 ml (1 tbsp) of sweet almond oil add 3 drops of chamomile or clary sage and 4 drops of orange, orange flower or petitgrain pure essence. Have a warm (but not too hot) bath, adding a few drops of one of the chosen essences, then use your oil preparation to massage your lower legs. With gentle but firm upward sweeps from your soles to above your knees, carry on massaging for at least 10 minutes, or until the oil is absorbed. Lie down for 30 minutes afterwards with your feet propped on a pillow or cushion, and inhale comforting lavender or one of the other essences from an oil burner.

- Build some regular exercise into your life. Gentle or brisk walking, dancing, skating, horse riding and ball games like tennis, table tennis and badminton all utilize your calf and upper leg muscles.

- Many practitioners of t'ai chi believe the slow graceful movements of this art/therapy are beneficial to restless legs.

- *Yoga* and Pilates, which strengthen and tone muscles without straining, are also helpful.

Drug remedies

○ The painkiller paracetamol or anti-inflammatory nurofen will give temporary relief.

○ Rutosides (bioflavonoids) are sometimes prescribed for poor circulation.

SEE YOUR DOCTOR IF...

- You experience any unexplained, involuntary leg movements.
- You have *varicose veins* or diabetes.

▪ Stroke

If you or someone close to you has had a stroke, you will know that the symptoms depend upon which area of the brain is affected. The underlying problem is ischaemia (loss of blood supply) brought about by clot formation, haemorrhage or an embolism.

A clot (or thrombus) forms in a brain artery clogged by fat, cutting off the circulation. If a brain artery bursts or leaks (cerebral haemorrhage), pressure builds up, the leaking stops and a clot forms. A brain embolism is a clot fragment from elsewhere in the body which lodges in a brain artery.

Whichever mechanism is involved, the resulting problems range from loss of consciousness, movement and speech to dizziness, confusion and heavy or numb limbs. Symptoms lasting 24 hours or longer mean that you have had a full stroke, but ones lasting just a few hours indicate a less severe mini-stroke or TIA (transient ischaemic attack).

Some strokes are preceded by a violent *headache* and nearly all are linked with furred-up, diseased arteries. *High blood pressure* and cholesterol greatly increase the risks of a stroke, but you can minimize these by the following measures.

WHAT YOU CAN DO

- Have regular blood pressure checks (SEE *High Blood Pressure*).

- Have regular cholesterol checks. If you have had raised cholesterol, your doctor will suggest dietary and lifestyle measures which can lower it naturally. If these are unsuccessful, take any medication as directed. If you experience side-effects, *don't* just stop – see your doctor for a change of prescription.

- Don't ignore 'funny turns' that may or may not be a TIA. The sooner a problem is identified, the sooner countermeasures can be taken.

- Stop smoking.

- Follow the rules for safe drinking. Binge drinking enormously increases the risks of a TIA or stroke.

- Nutritionally, the antioxidants in fresh, raw and puréed fruit and vegetables and their juices are helpful in boosting the strength of nervous tissue throughout the body and in helping brain and blood vessels to heal.

- All saturated fat should be replaced by polyunsaturates found in cold-pressed plant oils and their products.

- Choline, one of the B vitamins, emulsifies fat and helps to control cholesterol build-up. Found in egg yolks, green leafy vegetables, yeast, wheatgerm and liver, it works together with inositol, another B vitamin (found in cantaloupe melon, grapefruit, raisins, wheat germ, cabbage and peanuts). Both are important brain cell nutrients and are present in lecithin supplements available from health stores and pharmacies.

- A herbal treatment plan for a TIA or stroke would need to be drawn up by a qualified therapist in co-operation with your doctor, but ginseng (tea, capsules, etc.), lavender, oats and rosemary are all easily accessible restoratives for a debilitated central nervous system. Add essence of lavender or rosemary to bathwater or an oil burner and use rosemary in cooking.

Drug remedies

○ Various anti-coagulants (anti-clotting drugs) depending upon the type of stroke.

○ Aspirin and Persantin are prescribed alone or together after an initial TIA or stroke to prevent further attacks.

SEE YOUR DOCTOR IF...

- For regular BP and cholesterol checks.
- If you experience stroke-like symptoms or unusual episodes, for example reduced consciousness, heavy limb(s), difficulty with speech or movement, etc.
- You develop an uncustomary violent *headache*.

■ Varicose Veins

Potential varicose veins lie just below the skin of the lower limbs, draining into deep veins via interconnecting vessels. Blood in the deep vessels is encouraged to flow upwards by the massaging action of the surrounding leg muscles. Lack of exercise hampers this process; pressure builds up in the deep veins and is transmitted to the more vulnerable veins near the surface.

One-way valves help to prevent blood from pooling in the surface veins. However, some people are born with weak valves and prolonged back pressure damages them, overstretching their walls. Blue or purple bulges appear on the calf or thigh, and the legs ache and swell.

Varicose veins can easily be injured by minor cuts and scratches, and the thin overlying skin tends to bruise easily and tear. Due to the faulty circulation, an itchy rash – varicose *eczema* – or an ulcer can develop in the affected area.

WHAT YOU CAN DO

- Lose surplus weight and avoid putting on too much weight during pregnancy, which itself encourages varicose veins.

- Improve the blood flow in your deep leg veins by regular walking and other exercise. Go barefoot when possible or wear open sandals with moulded inner soles that encourage your toes to grip naturally to exercise your calf muscles.

- Put your feet up when you rest to encourage the blood to flow freely upwards.

- Wear elastic support stockings if recommended.

- A 13 cm (5 inches) block under the foot of your bed encourages nightly drainage of blood away from your legs.

- Guard against *constipation* (both straining and coughing increase the pressure within the abdomen and thereby the risks of vein disorders). Wholegrain flour products and five daily helpings of fresh fruit and vegetables supply fibre to keep the bowel active. Add figs, greengages, plums, rhubarb and their juices if extra help is required.

- Useful antioxidants for healthy blood vessels include vitamins A (beta carotene), B complex, C with bioflavonoids (especially hesperidin and rutin), D and E. Vitamin E relieves varicose vein inflammation (phlebitis) and helps to prevent it. You will find it in wholegrain cereals, soya beans, wheatgerm and its oil, egg yolks, cold pressed vegetable oil and spinach and other green leafy vegetables.

- You can also apply pure vitamin E oil or cream directly to inflamed veins, varicose *eczema* and varicose ulcers.

- Dab cider vinegar directly onto painful swollen veins or drink some to encourage weight loss. Take 15 mls (1 tbsp) of the (organic) vinegar three times daily, stirred into a tumbler of water.

- Clove essence added to pure cold water is sometimes used to bathe varicose *eczema* and ulcers. A common herbal prescription ointment is based on essences of benzoin and cypress, mixed with sweet almond oil and extracts of pure beeswax.

- Homoeopathic tincture of Hamamelis applied to painful varicose veins can bring rapid relief.

Drug remedies

○ There are no specific medicines for varicose veins, although the bioflavonoid extract oxerutins can relieve the swelling associated with them.

SEE YOUR DOCTOR IF...

- A varicose vein is injured – the profuse bleeding needs urgent medical attention.
- Your veins cause troublesome symptoms or you develop a rash or ulcer.
- You need help to lose weight.

11

Urinary and Genital Ailments

- Bartholin's abscess ● Cystitis ● Genital warts
- Heavy vaginal bleeding ● Menopausal problems
- Painful intercourse ● Painful penis ● Painful periods
- Potency problems ● Premenstrual syndrome
- Prostate gland enlargement ● Urethritis
- Urinary stones ● Vaginal discharge

■ Bartholin's Abscess

Bartholin's glands, on each side of the vulva close to the vaginal entrance, secrete lubricating fluid when you become sexually aroused. Blockage of a gland's opening by dirt or a plug of mucus traps the internal fluid, making the gland swell. The walls thicken, forming a Bartholin's cyst, and bacteria multiply inside, creating pus and a painful abscess.

The symptoms, which can come on suddenly, include soreness on one or other side of the vulva, which you notice during intercourse or when using lavatory paper. Soon, a throbbing pain starts and you can feel a tender lump in the vulva with your fingers. Sitting down can become very painful and you may develop *flu*-like symptoms such as a fever, *headache* and painful muscles as the infection becomes established.

WHAT YOU CAN DO

- Wash your vulval area thoroughly twice daily.

- Avoid tight-fitting jeans and underwear and thongs if you find they chafe you down below.

- Wear loose cool cotton skirts and pants, especially after sexual contact.

- Keep tiny specks of dirt away from your vulva. If outside, sit on a coat or rug.

- Shake sand and other debris out of pants and swimming costumes. Get your lover to wash their hands before sex, if they have been gardening or swimming.

- Boost your immunity with regular exercise and a healthy diet.

- Keep your fluid levels up with six to eight glasses of water daily (dehydration can lead to sticky secretions, which are more apt to clog glands). Juice carrots and apples together, adding a handful of fresh chervil leaves and several celery stalks, together with their tops. Sip up to 300 ml (½ pint) twice daily.

- Burdock root is a powerful immune-booster, anti-bacterial and anti-inflammatory, and medical herbalists often prescribe it in tablet form to cleanse the blood and encourage detoxification. It is a common ingredient in Japanese cuisine, which is noted for its healthy and energy-sustaining benefits.

- In Europe, fresh chervil is sometimes prescribed to treat *abscesses*. Make a hot compress or poultice using fresh chervil and apply it to the area.

- Take some paracetamol, either alone or combined with codeine, or a non-steroidal anti-inflammatory drug (NSAID) like ibuprofen or nurofen to relieve the pain and *flu*-like symptoms.

- Alternatively, make a warm oatmeal poultice (SEE *Herbal Medicine*), adding 4–5 drops of lavender, patchouli or tea tree essential oil, or soak in a long warm bath, adding a few drops of patchouli, rosemary or thuja essence, and/or inhale one or more of these by adding 3–4 drops to an oil burner.

- Drink some ginseng tea, prepared either from the fresh root or from a tea bag. Ginseng boosts immunity and, being an adaptogen (SEE *Herbal Medicine*), it helps to strengthen and stabilize your immune system when it is fighting infection.

Drug remedies

○ There are no specific drug remedies for Bartholin's abscess, but a little antiseptic cream applied to the area would have a soothing effect. Antibiotics are prescribed to overcome the bacterial infection.

SEE YOUR DOCTOR IF...

- You find any lump or swelling in or around your vulva. It needs to be identified, and a Bartholin's abscess treated with antibiotics, NSAIDs and/or other painkillers.

▪ Cystitis

If you're female, the chances are that you have had, or will have, cystitis (bladder inflammation) at some time. Men also suffer, although how they acquire it is more obscure. Most cystitis results from bacteria passing up the short female urethra (bladder outlet tube) and multiplying in the urine. The usual culprit is *E. coli*, found in the stools and transferred to the urethral opening from around the anus on lavatory paper, underwear, tampons and sexual intercourse.

When a cystitis attack starts, you may experience a scalding sensation on emptying your bladder, a sense of urgency when needing to go, passing a few drops at a time and feeling the need to pass more shortly afterwards. You may need to visit the bathroom several times during the night and your urine may be dark, bloodstained and/or offensive. If cystitis is ignored, the infection can spread up the ureters to the kidneys, causing *flu*-like symptoms such as fever, backache, *abdominal pain* and aches and pains in your limbs.

WHAT YOU CAN DO

- Use lavatory paper to wipe your bottom in a front to back direction. For recurrent cystitis, wash your perineum (between your legs) after opening your bowels. Pour cold boiled water from a bottle while sitting on the lavatory so that it washes over vulva and anus.

- Pass urine immediately after intercourse to rinse away any transferred germs.

- Take frequent baths and showers.

- Change tampons frequently.

- Wear loose cotton underwear and skirts instead of tight synthetic pants and trousers. Heat and perspiration encourage bacteria to breed.

- Drink six to eight tumblers of water daily. Cranberry juice and barley water are beneficial alternatives.

- Never keep a full bladder waiting! Stagnant urine is soon infected.

- Eat a wholefood diet with plenty of antioxidant-rich fresh fruit and vegetables to boost immunity. Celeriac, fennel, garlic and parsley are often recommended.

- Lavender tea is a traditional cystitis remedy. Add two to three fresh flowerheads or 5 ml (1 tsp) dried flowers to 560 ml (1 pint) of boiling water, infuse for 5 minutes, strain and sweeten with honey if desired. Sip several cups daily during an attack.

- Add three to four drops of *aromatherapy* essence of chamomile, eucalyptus, pine or sandalwood and/or inhale cajeput, cedarwood or niauoli in steam or from an oil burner. Make a hot compress with any of these oils and apply to your lower tummy while resting.

- Try a homoeopathic remedy every 30 minutes for up to ten doses:

  o For burning, cutting pain in the lower abdomen, a constant need to urinate, *lower backache* which is worse in the afternoon and only a trickle of bloodstained urine passed: Cantheris 30c

  o For a high fever, severe pain in the bladder, which is hard and swollen, restlessness and agitation: Tarantula 6c

  o For cystitis symptoms triggered by sexual intercourse or after a catheter has been passed for medical reasons, a constant burning sensation even when not urinating and a urethra which feels as though a drop of urine is continually passing down it: Staphisagria 6c

Drug remedies

○ Painkillers such as paracetamol, aspirin or NSAIDs (non-steroidal anti-inflammatory drugs such as ibuprofen or nurofen).

○ Antibiotics – e.g. ciprofloxacin, nalidixuc acid, nitrofurantoin, trimethoprim.

○ Effervescent potassium citrate tablets to alkalize the urine.

SEE YOUR DOCTOR IF...

• Your bladder symptoms do not subside within 24 hours.
• You develop a fever, backache or other signs of kidney infection.
• Your urine is discoloured or smelly.
• Home remedies do not help.

▪ Genital Warts

Genital warts are small pink finger-like growths in and around the vulva and penis and sometimes around the anus. They vary from minute nodules to 1 cm (½ inch) in length and are caused by a virus, some strains of which are known to increase the risk of cervical cancer. Itching and irritation occur, and the warts can bleed if scratched. They then smart and sting after intercourse and when in contact with urine.

Following treatment, the wart virus can remain dormant, then break out again if your immune system becomes weakened. This can also happen when your vaginal secretions are increased by pregnancy or thrush or a similar infection. Genital warts are moderately contagious and easily passed on by sexual contact; they can also spread from warts elsewhere on the body (SEE *Warts*).

WHAT YOU CAN DO

- Always use condoms with new sexual partners. (Do not assume because your partner is wart-free that they are not carrying the wart virus.)

- Have regular cervical smears.

- Avoid sex at any time if you or your partner's genital area is red and sore.

- Boost your immunity (SEE *Nutritional Medicine*) and drink some vitamin C-rich juices daily. You could make a fruit salad juice with several citrus fruits, honey if needed, blueberries, raspberries and cherries. Zinc helps your body to fight infection – you will find this in lean meat, wheatgerm, eggs, pumpkin seeds and mustard powder and seeds.

- Squeeze some juice from two to three fresh garlic cloves and apply this twice daily to the warts. Celandine cream is also said to help.

- The essential oil of bay (*Laurus nobilis*) has anti-viral properties. It is best used under the guidance of a qualified aromatherapist (who might also/alternatively prescribe the highly potent oil of gaiac, also called *Lignum vitae* or tree of life), but you can still add a drop or two of bay essence to your bathwater or inhale it from an oil burner. If you like the flavour, add bay leaves to soups and casseroles, pilau rice and other vegetable and grain dishes, and to rice pudding (remove the leaves before eating).

- Stress depletes immunity, so practise deep *relaxation*, *Yoga* and meditation. Warts are traditionally linked to charm cures, so you may benefit from positive *autohypnosis*. When fully relaxed, spend 10 minutes daily concentrating on your warts and repeating suitable words such as 'My warts are shrinking and will soon be gone.' *Visualize this happening...*

Drug remedies

○ Podophyllotoxin solution, applied directly to *external* warts with an applicator provided twice daily for 3 days and repeated if necessary at weekly intervals (i.e. 4 days later) for up to 5 weeks.

○ Imiquimod cream, applied directly to *external* warts 3 times weekly at bedtime for up to 16 weeks.

○ Inosine prabonex tablets (SEE *below*).

SEE YOUR DOCTOR IF...

• You develop lumps, swellings or growths of any sort in the genital and/or anal region.

• You have warts inside the vaginal lips. These can be treated with a carbon dioxide laser and anti-viral inosine prabonex tablets prescribed if required.

• Have an annual cervical smear if your partner suffers from genital warts or if you have done so in the past.

■ Heavy Vaginal Bleeding

If you suffer from unusually heavy periods, you might have prolonged frequent bleeds or a heavy loss for a week or so each month. What is counted as 'heavy' is generally subjective, but doctors look for flooding (blood soaking tampons, towels and underclothes) and anaemia when making a diagnosis. The causes include hormonal imbalance, fibroids, endometriosis, pelvic inflammatory disease (PID), the coil contraceptive and the contraceptive injection.

Fibroids and polyps cause painless heavy blood loss. Both are non-malignant growths in the womb lining and can be removed by surgery – a hysterectomy may be suggested for large multiple fibroids, especially if you have no further wish for children. Endometriosis, where the womb lining cells are deposited elsewhere, such as the womb walls, bladder, colon or rectum, could be the cause if your heavy bleeding is accompanied by *painful intercourse* and severe cramping period pains (SEE *Painful Periods*).

PID often results from a vaginal infection which has spread to the pelvic organs. Besides heavy and/or irregular bleeding, you might develop low *abdominal pain*, cramping, an offensive *vaginal discharge*, nausea, fever and *cystitis*-like symptoms.

WHAT YOU CAN DO

- Keep a diary of blood loss days, the number of tampons or towels used, clots passed and other symptoms.

- If you use the coil or have progesterone injections, a different form of contraception may help.

- Seek medical help promptly for a persistent/offensive *vaginal discharge* to prevent infection spreading to the pelvis.

- A wholefood diet boosts your stamina, combats anaemia and helps to rectify minor hormonal imbalances. Include daily helpings of fresh fruit and vegetables, and sources of iron – wholemeal-enriched bread, cheddar cheese, egg yolk, chickpeas, molasses (black treacle), lentils and walnuts.

- A naturopathic diet often recommended for heavy periods caused by fibroids or endometriosis includes 1 g of protein per kilo (1 oz per 66 lbs) of body weight per day. Its aim is to reduce the adverse effects of oestrogen in the body and hasten the liver's conversion of naturally produced oestrogens into the less harmful oestradiol. Good protein sources include fat-free organic red meat and offal, pulses, grains, seeds and nuts.

- Sip some fresh carrot juice daily – its beta-carotene content helps you to maximize the benefits of dietary iron. Vitamin C helps you absorb iron – try freshly squeezed orange juice alone or mixed 1:1 with canned or packet tomato juice.

- Add 2–3 drops of cypress essential oil to your bath or inhale it from an oil burner.

- Homoeopathic remedies to be taken every 8 hours for up to ten doses, starting just before your period is due:

  o For intermittent bleeding, black blood clots, faintness, *dizzy spells*, a pale face and cramping pains: China 30c

  o For nausea with heavy loss of bright red blood: Ipecac 30c

  o For flooding, dark watery blood, a pale face, occasional flushes, improved by walking about: Ferrum 30c

Drug remedies

o The NSAID mefenamic acid or the anti-haemorrhagic drug tranexamic acid are prescribed for heavy periods.

o When contraception is required, the combined oral contraceptive pill is often effective. Norethisterone, a long-acting progestogen, is sometimes chosen.

SEE YOUR DOCTOR IF...

- You experience persistently heavy bleeding.
- Home remedies do not help.

▪ Menopausal Problems

Menopausal problems mean different things to different women. Perhaps intercourse has become painful, your vagina feels dry and sore and your interest in love-making has waned. Or you may experience *urethritis* and need to pass urine more frequently, especially at night. Alternatively, hot flushes and night sweats might be plaguing you at work, when socializing or when stressed, angry or tired. Some sufferers experience the whole symptom spectrum which, in addition to the above, includes mood swings, irritability and *depression*, loss of concentration and memory, poor self-esteem and one or more fractured bones.

The underlying problem is the reduction in blood oestrogen which takes place when your ovaries have finished shedding their eggs and you are no longer ovulating. The superficial veins in the skin are affected, causing sweats and flushes. The vaginal and urethral linings – both influenced by oestrogen – start to thin and age, and can become inflamed. It's common to feel more tired than usual during the change and to lose self-confidence – partly because your mood is low anyway and partly because the symptoms can make you feel old, useless and sexually unattractive.

WHAT YOU CAN DO

- Wholefoods with five or more daily helpings of fresh fruit and vegetables and their juices supply antioxidants which boost immunity and help to retard the ageing process. Low-GI carbohydrates (SEE *Nutritional Medicine*) reduce the risk of hypoglycaemia (low blood sugar) which often results from a diet high in sugar and other refined carbohydrates (SEE *Blood Sugar Imbalance*). Cutting back on junk and processed foods also encourages weight loss.

- Take soya products regularly for their phytoestrogen content (or a supplement of these natural substances).

- Exercise to maintain physical fitness. Non-arduous weight training (in the gym or at home) improves muscular strength. Brisk walking, swimming, dancing, horse-riding and other forms of exercise that increase your pulse rate and make you perspire a little combat a low mood, release tension and tone the heart and lungs.

- Exercise involving foot contact with the ground strengthens bones against the thinning disease osteoporosis and reduces the risk of fractures.

- Stretching exercises keep your muscles and joints flexible and supple and help to maintain your co-ordination. Try something new – *Yoga*, t'ai chi and Pilates are excellent choices.

- Establish inner calm! Take up *Yoga* and regular *relaxation*, meditate and/or listen to soothing music. Have a regular massage, start a new hobby. Studies confirm that the busier and more involved you remain, the less likely you are to experience menopausal problems.

- Use aloe vera liquid or gel to lubricate and soothe vaginal dryness.

- Herbal remedies containing helonias root, agnus castus, oats, St John's wort, life root and the relaxants chamomile and black haw can all prove helpful.

- Add *aromatherapy* essence of rose to your bath or oil burner to increase self-confidence, especially about personal attractiveness. Rose also has aphrodisiac properties. Rose and geranium both ease menopausal symptoms, while chamomile dispels irritability and improves sleep.

- Homoeopathic remedies to take every 12 hours for up to 7 days:

  o For hot flushes, sweating, tense stomach, light-headedness, morning *headaches*, flooding, being very talkative: Lachesis 30c

  o For a dry vagina, *constipation* and black burned-looking stools: Bryonia 30c

- Try the *Bach Flower Remedy* Hornbeam if you are weary and cannot cope, or Gorse for feelings of despair and that there is no point in trying.

Drug remedies

o Hormone replacement therapy (HRT) can be prescribed but recent studies have linked it with an increased risk of breast cancer and more women are turning to natural hormone substitutes, derived from plant sources.

SEE YOUR DOCTOR IF...

- Home remedies do not work.
- You experience persistent and troublesome symptoms.

▪ Painful Intercourse

If you're finding intercourse painful, you'll want to know why and how to relieve it. If you are a woman, muscle spasm, pelvic inflammation, infection (SEE *Vaginal Discharge*) and thinning vaginal membranes (SEE *Menopausal Problems*) can all be responsible (SEE ALSO *Potency Problems, Painful Penis*). Penetration becomes difficult if you are insufficiently aroused, nervous or tense. You could need more foreplay, a gentler technique or simply the strength to say no if you are tired or off-colour.

Vaginismus is common in young women during their first sexual encounters. Anxiety and tension cause the muscles of the pelvis and thighs to clamp down, making penetration impossible. Symptoms suggesting a possible medical cause include heavy or irregular periods, *abdominal pain, vaginal discharge* and fever. Endometriosis, in which cells from the womb lining are found elsewhere in the pelvis, and an ovarian cyst can also be responsible.

WHAT YOU CAN DO

- If you are anxious and tense, discuss personal worries with a parent, sister or friend, and safe sex and contraceptive choices with your GP or Family Planning Clinic doctor.

- Remember that vaginismus is *common* and can be successfully treated. *Never* try to force penetration, which can only cause physical and emotional scars.

- Stay fit and active with a healthy wholefood diet. Drink six- to eight glasses of water daily and eat lots of fresh fruit and vegetables supplying antioxidants. Calming, invigorating juices include lettuce, celery and small quantities of spinach, mixed with apple or carrot.

- Try calming herbal teas such as chamomile, melissa or mint or orange blossom and a long relaxing bath before bed.

- Use regular gentle exercise to release stress. *Yoga*, with its deep breathing exercises and slow calm stretching is a wonderful *relaxation* aid. It also tones the muscles of the pelvis and around the vagina and improves their flexibility. Beneficial asanas might include the Cobra, Fish, Plough and Uddiyana.

- Suitable *Bach Flower Remedies* could include Mimulus (for fear of specific known things, for example pain, and for shy, nervous people), and Aspen, for trembling apprehension and vague unidentified fears.

- *Aromatherapy* rose oil is especially beneficial for female intercourse problems, because it promotes sexual self-confidence. Add a few drops to your bathwater or to 15 ml (1 tbsp) of sweet almond oil and use it as a pelvic massage oil. You can also inhale rose oil, or the tranquillizing essences of cedarwood, clove, lavender or ylang ylang from an oil burner.

- Homoeopathic remedies may help. Take these every 12 hours for up to 5 days:

  - For a woman who is very emotional and tearful, often blushes and dislikes hot stuffy rooms: Pulsatilla 30c

  - For difficulties caused by grief or disappointment in an earlier relationship: Ignatia 30c

- And try these every 4 hours for up to 2 weeks:

  - For when the vagina is extra sensitive, with stabbing pain in the left side of the pelvis after intercourse: Thuja 6c

  - For a hypersensitive genital area, with cystitis brought on by love-making or pain in one or other side of the pelvis during love-making: Staphisagria 6c

Drug remedies

- Antiseptic creams are used to treat minor irritations around the vaginal opening.

- KY jelly supplies useful lubrication.

SEE YOUR DOCTOR IF...

- Simple home remedies do not help.
- You have vaginismus – plastic dilators can be prescribed to widen a small vagina.
- Intercourse starts to become painful without explanation.

▪ Painful Penis

If the head of your penis and foreskin become inflamed (balanitis), common causes include soiled, damp or rough underpants and grains of dirt between your foreskin and penile head. Infections, including thrush, can develop, especially if you are diabetic, because the urine's high glucose content encourages bacteria to multiply.

If intercourse is painful, your partner's vagina may be too dry, and if your penis becomes inflamed afterwards, you could be sensitive to chemicals in condoms, the contraceptive cap or spermicidal creams.

Painful erections are sometimes due to phimosis – difficulty in drawing back the foreskin over the head of the penis. It is generally diagnosed in babies and small children, but it can become a problem during puberty when erections start.

Genital herpes is usually to blame for painful open sores and *genital warts* appear as small tough growths. Both will cause you discomfort and interfere with love-making. Any inflammation of the penile tip can spread inside the urethra, causing a scalding sensation on passing urine.

WHAT YOU CAN DO

- Wash your genital area twice daily, pulling back the foreskin to remove perspiration or dirt.

- Encourage air to circulate with cool loose cotton underpants worn clean daily.

- Eliminate any chemicals that may be producing an allergy.

- If your partner suffers from vaginal dryness, spend longer on foreplay and use lubricating KY jelly or aloe vera gel.

- If she has thrush and you haven't been circumcised, apply Canesten cream to the head of your penis for a fortnight (and use condoms throughout this period).

- Five or more daily helpings of fresh fruit and vegetables and their juices supply the vitamins, minerals, trace elements and anti-oxidants your immune system needs to combat allergy and infection.

- Morning Eye-Opener contains vitamin C and bioflavonoids (among others) which help to heal damaged membranes. Juice fresh oranges to make a good 300 ml (½ pint), add the juice of 1 lime and 1 lemon, and 5–10 ml (1–2 tsp) of the finely grated zest from one or more of the fruit. Stir in a heaped dessertspoon of organic comb honey and the contents of 2 capsules of royal jelly and 2 of pollen. Serve over ice cubes with fresh mint or lemon thyme sprigs.

- Herbal preparations of celery, saw palmetto and gravelroot all soothe inflamed urinary mucous membranes and combat infection.

- Look for any sore areas and apply an antiseptic cream, for example Savlon, or one containing calendula and hypericum extract, for example Nelson's Hypercal.

- Inhale essential oil of juniper using an oil burner, or add 4–5 drops to bathwater and have a good soak.

- Try the following homoeopathic remedies:

  o For balanitis, to take 4 hourly for up to 5 days: Mercurius 6c

  o For penile *warts*, to take four times daily for up to 14 days: remedy of first resort: Thuja 6c; if there is no improvement with Thuja, and if your *warts* bleed easily and your foreskin is swollen: Cinnabar 6c

  o For sexual difficulties linked to the *warts*, for example premature ejaculation or erectile problems: Lycopodium 6c

Drug remedies

o Antiseptic creams, for example those containing cetrimide, chlorhexidine, for balanitis.

o Antibiotic creams may be necessary for infected balanitis.

o KY jelly or aloe vera liquid or gel to improve vaginal penetration.

SEE YOUR DOCTOR IF...

- You develop *any* sores, small growths, lumps, etc. on or around the penis.
- Home remedies do not help.

▪ Painful Periods

Periods can be painful from the time they start during puberty, but often for a year or so produce no symptoms other than vaginal bleeding. Once you start to ovulate, though, you may experience typical period pain deep down in the lower tummy and/or the back. The long cramping spasms, which can be severe, often start a day or so before the bleeding and may put you out of action for a few hours, although it is generally best to try to keep going.

You might also feel sick or faint, develop a *headache* and become miserable and touchy (SEE ALSO *Premenstrual Syndrome*). Painful periods that start early in life are known medically as primary dysmenorrhoea. They can be distressing, but they are not abnormal and they become less troublesome as the years pass. You are likely to notice a huge improvement after having your first baby.

Secondary dysmenorrhoea, starting in later life, is usually due to an underlying condition like fibroids, endometriosis or PID (SEE *Vaginal Discharge*), which needs to be diagnosed and treated.

WHAT YOU CAN DO

- Eat wholefoods with plenty of fresh vegetables and fruit (eaten raw or lightly cooked wherever possible), plus eggs, poultry, fish, grains, pulses and/or nuts as sources of protein and low-GI carbohydrates (SEE *Nutritional Medicine*).

- Period pains are aggravated by *constipation*, so keep regular with the above high-fibre foods of your choice.

- Dietary supplements of ferrous gluconate (easily absorbed iron), folic acid and pollen are said to be very helpful. Add some royal jelly (a natural product of queen bees) and/or evening primrose oil (SEE *Premenstrual Syndrome*).

- Exercise helps! The pain is partly due to congestion of the walls of your uterus (womb) and walking, skating, dancing and horse-riding all tone the pelvic and back muscles, relieving pelvic congestion. They also encourage your bowels to work regularly. When moderate to severe pain is present, however, you are better off lying completely still.

- Depending on your symptoms, helpful herbal remedies could include agnus castus, blue cohosh, black cohosh and black haw.

- Exercise also provides an escape valve for pent-up emotions and mild *depression*. Even when feeling down, a brisk walk in the fresh air will make you feel calmer and more cheerful.

- If pelvic pain and *headache* do get the upper hand, take a paracetamol or some nurofen and lie down with a hot water bottle against your lower tummy or back. Chew some crystallized ginger to ward off nausea or sip some ginger or chamomile tea.

- Try these homoeopathic remedies hourly for up to ten doses:

  - For pain that is worst immediately before your period, with a dragging sensation aggravated by lying down, and when the blood is bright red and your skin is flushed and burning: Belladonna 30c

  - For severe cramping pains similar to labour pain, with *headaches* before the period starts: Cimicifuga 30c

  - For late scanty periods causing pain extending to the thighs: Viburnum 30c

  - For severe cramps, especially when there is a feeling of rage and extreme restlessness: Chamomilla 30c

Drug remedies

- Painkillers such as paracetamol, nurofen or ibuprofen and muscle relaxants such as hyoscine (Buscopan) prove useful to many sufferers.

- The contraceptive pill is sometimes prescribed to suppress ovulation for a few months, thereby relieving the painful spasms.

SEE YOUR DOCTOR IF...

- Simple home remedies fail to relieve your symptoms.
- You suffer from *fainting attacks*, severe *headaches*, vomiting or other troublesome symptoms.

■ Potency Problems

Potency problems range from difficulty in obtaining or maintaining an erection to an inability to ejaculate during climax. Traditionally, men have been (understandably though unnecessarily) embarrassed by this common disorder, although the arrival of Viagra and similar drugs is now encouraging more sufferers to seek medical advice, knowing that help is available.

One variation of potency difficulty is achieving a partial erection, but with the penis remaining too limp and floppy for penetration. Another is getting an erection during foreplay, only for it to disappear when you attempt intercourse. Yet another is finding the process uncomfortable, with shooting pains in the penis and/or testicles when attempting to make love. Any one or combination of these can make you so fearful of 'failures' that your sex urge is desperately low. *Depression* also depletes libido and antidepressants (among other drugs) can interfere with erection.

Reduced blood supply to the genitals is a common cause of impotence or semi-impotence in middle-aged or diabetic men and in others with fat-clogged arteries. (For *arterial clogging*, SEE *Angina* and *Poor Circulation in the Feet*.)

WHAT YOU CAN DO

- A wholefood diet with plenty of fresh fruit and vegetables is a must for renewed vigour, stamina and sexual performance.

Oily fish, lean meat, eggs, poultry, soya foods, grains, pulses, legumes and nuts provide carbohydrates and proteins for energy and cell renewal. Cold-pressed vegetable oils rich in cis-linoleic acid encourage the production of prostaglandins E1, needed for the control of male and female sexual function (SEE *Premenstrual Syndrome* and *Drug Remedies*).

- Freshly squeezed red cabbage, celery and lettuce juices are recommended for potency problems.

- Exercise to release tension.

- Learn to relax.

- Beat negative emotions with an appropriate *Bach Flower Remedy*.

- Sandalwood *aromatherapy* essence does for male sexual desire and confidence what Rose essence does for female. Add 5–6 drops to 20 ml (4 tsp) sweet almond oil and share a massage with your partner.

- Try these *acupressure* points:

  ○ Bigger Stream

  ○ Bubbling Springs

  ○ Three Mile Point – to increase stamina and boost the sexual organs

Drug remedies

○ Sildenafil (Viagra), tadalafil (Cialis) and vardenafil, available as tablets, all work by increasing the blood flow to the penis and enhancing the response to sexual stimulation.

○ Alprostadil (an E1 prostaglandin, SEE *Premenstrual Syndrome*) is given by self-administered injection into the penis or through the urethra.

o Apomorphine, available as tablets to be placed under the tongue, works on brain centres and nerve pathways to produce an erection within 20 minutes.

SEE YOUR DOCTOR IF...

- You are depressed or suffer from *anxiety* or mood swings (or have done so in the past).
- You take regular medication – this needs checking for side-effects.
- Simple home remedies do not work.

■ Premenstrual Syndrome (PMS)

Also known as PMT, or premenstrual tension, PMS is a group of physical and emotional ailments which can affect you from between a day to a fortnight before your period starts. Common symptoms include bloating, weight gain, tender breasts and *headaches*, mood swings, feeling blue, tense and irritable, poor memory and concentration.

PMS has been widely studied since the early 1980s and suggested causes include food sensitivity, nutritional factors, for example calcium and magnesium metabolism, and hormonal imbalances.

A major trigger may be the failure of a cellular enzyme to convert the essential omega-6 fatty acids (found in cold-pressed unprocessed plant oils) into the active substance gamma-linolenic acid (GLA). You need GLA in order to manufacture short-lived hormone-like prostaglandins (PGs) which control the normal functioning of sexual and other organs. Inadequate levels of the E1 group of prostaglandins are believed to make some women hyper-sensitive to minor (i.e. normal) variations in hormone levels in the second half of their cycle, producing PMS symptoms.

WHAT YOU CAN DO

- Follow a wholefood diet with plenty of fresh vegetables and fruit, eating as much raw as possible. Reduce your fat intake, especially the saturated (animal) type. Cut down on salt, junk snacks and convenience foods and on processed plant oils and their products, for example margarines. Commercial manufacture changes vital cis-fatty acids into the harmful 'trans' variety, which interfere with prostaglandin production. Cold-pressed vegetable oils supply cis-linoleic acid naturally. Safflower, sunflower, olive, corn oil are all good choices. Use them once only for frying – reheated oil is full of trans-acids.

- If you are prone to hypoglycaemia (low blood sugar), which causes faintness, sweating, a racing pulse and shakiness and is linked to PMS, it is especially important to avoid sugary snacks and high-GI carbohydrates (SEE *Blood Sugar Imbalance* and *Nutritional Medicine*).

- Instead of one or two large daily meals, eat small frequent snacks of raw fruit or vegetables and their juices, low-GI carbohydrates and protein.

- Take a multivitamin/mineral supplement, or at least vitamins B6, C and E, magnesium and zinc – all required for PG production from cis-linoleic acid and GLA. Take a calcium supplement, too.

- Take an evening primrose oil supplement, starting a day or so each month before your symptoms usually start. Useful herbal remedies (depending upon your particular problem) include agnus castus and blue flag.

- Take some regular exercise to boost your mood and release tension (SEE *Painful Periods*). Try *Yoga*, deep *relaxation* and/or meditation for their harmonizing effects.

- Useful *Bach Flower Remedies* might include Beech, Gentian, for a low mood, Holly and Impatiens.

- Geranium and rosemary essential oils combat fluid retention – add 3–4 drops to your bath or inhale from an oil burner. Chamomile, lavender and marjoram oil all soothe *lower backache* or abdominal cramps. Add 2–3 drops to 10 ml (1 dsp) sweet almond oil and massage gently into your lower abdomen or back.

Drug remedies

o Painkillers for stomachache, backache and headache (SEE *Painful Periods*).

o A supplement of the hormone progesterone in tablet form or as a vaginal pessary.

o Diuretic drugs such as bendroflumethiazide (water pills) may be prescribed for fluid retention. You can buy herbal diuretics from pharmacies and health food stores.

o Sometimes an antidepressant can help (SEE *Depression*).

SEE YOUR DOCTOR IF...

- PMS symptoms are making you/others miserable.
- You suffer from severe mood swings.
- Your aggression is uncontrollable and unpredictable – you feel a threat to yourself or others.
- Simple home treatments do not bring relief.

▪ Prostate Gland Enlargement

The male prostate gland surrounds the neck of the bladder and the upper part of its outlet tube, the urethra. Its secretions form part of the semen released during climax. From early middle age the gland tends to enlarge, nipping the urethra passing through it. This is BPH, or benign prostatic hypertrophy – non-cancerous prostate gland enlargement – and it can cause some irritating symptoms. You will need to pass water more frequently, yet often feel that your bladder never really empties. You may have a feeble urine flow and lose some control over starting and stopping the stream. You may be embarrassed by 'terminal dribbling', i.e. a leakage of urine onto your underpants after you have 'finished'. And you may have to strain to force the last few drops out. Your sleep is likely to be disturbed by nightly trips to the bathroom and outings may become a problem because of your constant need to be in reach of a lavatory.

WHAT YOU CAN DO

- A wholefood diet and range of supplements can help to relieve BPH symptoms.

- *Don't* drink less fluid because passing it is problematical – you will only become dehydrated. Drink six to eight glasses of water a day and avoid caffeine-containing drinks like coffee, tea and cola because they can cause urethral irritation.

- Freshly squeezed carrot, beetroot and cucumber juices in roughly equal proportions are recommended. Start with 300 ml (½ pint) once or twice daily and increase as you wish.

- A regular intake of fresh fruit and vegetables can itself be beneficial because of the natural hormone-like substances many contain. Make sure you include fresh and cooked tomatoes daily.

- Increase your intake of zinc – a nutrient the gland badly needs. Look for it in organic lamb, eggs, wheatgerm, pumpkin seeds, fat-free milk powder and powdered mustard. Alternatively (or in addition), take a multivitamin/mineral supplement and some zinc gluconate.

- Pollen (available as capsules and tablets) is clinically proven to reduce prostate gland swelling and the associated symptoms.

- Cranberry extracts and juice ease a sore, sensitive bladder and reduce the risks of urinary infection.

- Saw palmetto has a specific hormonal action on the male reproductive organs and reduces BPH.

- Make a warm or cool compress using essential oil of lavender, or add 3–4 drops to 10 ml (1 dsp) sweet almond oil and massage your lower abdomen and perineal region (between your testicles and anus).

- Try these homoeopathic remedies four times daily for up to 21 days:

  o For difficulty or pain on trying to empty the bladder and spasms of bladder pain: Sabal 6c

  o For someone who is senile and who urinates a lot at night, complains of pressure in the rectum and smarting sensation inside the bladder: Ferrum pic. 6c

  o For a frequent urge to urinate, producing a slow stream, especially if underweight, thin and impotent: Baryta 6c

Drug remedies

  o The drug finasteride reduces the risks of acute urinary retention, a painful and distressing condition in which you can pass no urine at all. It also reduces your chances of needing an operation.

○ Doxazosin and similar drugs are also prescribed to relieve the restricted urinary flow and other symptoms of BPH.

SEE YOUR DOCTOR IF...

- You develop *any* symptoms you think may be due to your prostate gland. A diagnosis is essential to rule out cancer or other causes.
- Your symptoms worsen or remain troublesome despite home treatments.

■ Urethritis

Urethritis – inflammation of the urethra or bladder outlet tube – has some symptoms in common with *cystitis*, but local irritants are more often to blame than infection, at least in women. You notice a burning sensation when you empty your bladder and you need to 'go' more frequently. If the urethra is very inflamed, your urine may be pink-tinged with blood. The absence of low tummy and back pain, fever, tenderness over your bladder and dark smelly urine are all reasons to consider possible urethritis triggers, rather than *cystitis*, and eliminate them one by one.

An evening's heavy drinking can cause urethritis while the waste products of alcohol are being excreted in your urine. Other dietary factors include highly spiced food, strong coffee and tea, cola drinks, beans, onions and chocolate. Extremes of temperature and sitting around in wet swimming clothes can also bring on an attack. Vigorous intercourse and the overuse of vibrators can bruise the lining of the urethra, which then becomes inflamed. Condoms can cause chemical irritation, as can oils and perfumes added to bathwater.

Urethritis in men is often – although not invariably – caused by a genital infection for which medical treatment should be sought.

WHAT YOU CAN DO

- Drink lots of water – dehydration concentrates the urine and therefore any chemical irritants it may contain.

- Avoid or take less of any foods/drinks which may be acting as triggers.

- Take a change of swimwear to wear by the pool or on the beach after you have finished in the water.

- Don't perch on hot radiators or sit on the cold damp ground.

- If you're a woman, sitting in a bath of warm or tepid water should immediately relieve the symptoms.

- Avoid scented soaps, bath oils and talcum powder, and vaginal deodorants.

- Ask your partner to be extra gentle when making love. Irritation from condoms and spermicidal creams may mean choosing a different form of contraception.

- Follow a wholefood diet with plenty of fresh fruit and vegetables rich in antioxidants.

- Freshly squeezed carrot juice mixed with the same volume of celery or apple juice is a recognized urethritis remedy.

- Make a cold perineal compress by adding 2–3 drops of niaouli or pine essential oil to a small bowl of iced water. Soak a clean cloth, wring it out and apply it as close to your urethral opening as you can. Refresh as necessary.

- Try a homoeopathic remedy every 30 minutes for up to ten doses:

  - For an attack that starts after getting damp and cold after exertion, especially in the autumn, with bloodstained urine which you need to pass often: Dulcamara 6c

○ For when the urine stream is slow and intermittent: Clematis 6c

○ For a burning pain inside the urethra whenever you urinate and an urgency to pass urine which has a thick and slightly opaque appearance: Sarsaparilla 6c

Drug remedies

○ There are no specific drug remedies for non-infective urethritis, although effervescent potassium citrate tablets to alkalize the urine and NSAIDs (non-steroidal anti-inflammatory drugs) such as those mentioned for *cystitis* might provide some relief.

SEE YOUR DOCTOR IF...

- You develop full-blown *cystitis* symptoms.
- The problem persists despite home treatments.

▪ Urinary Stones

If you have suffered from kidney stones (renal calculus), you will know the distress they can cause. The symptoms include a dull pain in your loin to the side of the spine, just below your ribs, and blood or pus in the urine. Renal colic develops when a kidney stone or fragment passes into the ureter leading to your bladder and gets stuck. The muscular walls of this tube squeeze vigorously to overcome the obstruction, causing spasms from loin to groin which can spread into the testicle or the outer vagina and the inner thighs. The pain can be agonizing and you may go into shock with a racing pulse, pallor, sweating and vomiting. Renal colic stops when the stone is expelled into the bladder, but if untreated, it can continue for several days.

There are different varieties of renal stone (SEE *below*) and a major trigger is stagnant infected urine (due to the bladder not emptying properly), which allows waste solids to accumulate. Others include drinking too little fluid (which concentrates the urine, encouraging stone formation) and raised urinary levels of calcium or uric acid.

WHAT YOU CAN DO

- Concentrated urine gives rise to stones, so drink 2 litres (3½ pints) of water daily.

- Go easy on dairy products – an unusually high intake could encourage calcium stone formation.

- You have an increased risk of urate stones if you are a gout sufferer, so have your blood uric acid levels checked regularly. Gout involves a problem with purine metabolism, so limit your intake of purine-rich foods such as bouillon, meat extracts, offal, yeast, anchovies, herrings, sardines and fish roe.

- Thiazide diuretics (water pills) prescribed for fluid retention and *high blood pressure* can also raise blood uric acid. Check which type you are on if you have had stones in the past.

- Do not postpone emptying your bladder – stagnant urine soon becomes infected and stones easily form. If you're a man experiencing difficulty in passing urine, ask your doctor to check your prostate gland (SEE *Prostate Gland Enlargement*). Medication can be prescribed to help you empty your bladder more easily.

- Boost your immune defences against infection – follow a wholefood diet rich in fresh fruit and vegetables and their juices.

Beetroot, carrot and cucumber in equal proportions are claimed to dissolve renal stones – sip between ½–1 litre (1–2 pints) daily.

- Holistic nutritionists sometimes prescribe defatted rice bran to treat an abnormally high level of calcium in the urine (this can be a symptom of disordered parathyroid glands, and you would doubtless be receiving conventional treatment too).

- To relieve painful spasms, add 5–6 drops of borage oil to 20 ml (2 dsp) almond oil and use to massage your lower abdomen (with clockwise strokes) and loin area.

Drug remedies

○ There is no specific drug treatment for kidney stones, but an opiate painkiller such as morphine or pethidine might be given by intramuscular injection or by mouth to treat acute symptoms or to a patient awaiting surgery.

○ An opiate-related drug such as fentanyl or tramadol, or an NSAID such as ibuprofen with, for example, a paracetamol + codeine combination might be prescribed for a patient being investigated for recurrent renal colic.

SEE YOUR DOCTOR IF...

- *Urgently* if you experience severe pain or any of the symptoms of shock.
- You are suffering from renal stone symptoms and home treatments do not help.
- You notice or suspect blood or pus in your urine.

▪ Vaginal Discharge

A transparent odourless vaginal discharge mid-cycle or just before your period and slight vaginal bleeding when you ovulate mid-cycle are both normal. A smelly discharge and painful intercourse, however, suggest a vaginal infection.

Thrush, caused by the *Candida* fungus (SEE *Intestinal Thrush*), produces a thick white discharge with a yeasty smell. It's intensely itchy and your vagina and vulva become red and sore. *Trichomonas* gives you a heavy greenish bubbly discharge with a fishy smell. Untreated, it can cause pelvic inflammatory disease (PID). The discharge from *Gardnerella* also smells fishy, but it is watery, thin and heavier mid-cycle and after sex.

A yellow discharge starting within seven days of unprotected sex, plus a sore vulva and vagina and having to pass water more frequently, suggests gonorrhoea. This can also cause PID and infertility. It is often found together with *Chlamydia*, which gives you a bloodstained discharge, deep pelvic pain and fever, although it can take some time for symptoms to appear. Neglected, *Chlamydia* gives rise to PID and infertility, and can harm your unborn baby.

WHAT YOU CAN DO

- Practise safe sex – use a condom.

- Beware with whom you share – *Trichomonas*, for example, though usually transmitted sexually, can occasionally be caught from a dirty lavatory seat or from another person's face cloth, towel, pants or swimming costume. Ask your partner to have a health check: men can carry STDs (sexually transmitted diseases) without experiencing symptoms.

- Boost your immunity – *Trichomonas* and *Candida* are commonly found in the vagina, vulva, bladder and anus, and develop into infections only when you are run down or when the balance of helpful bacteria is reduced by, for example, antibiotics.

- Eat five or more portions of fresh fruit and vegetables daily, preferably raw or lightly cooked. A 1:1 mixture of celery and carrot juice helps increase your resistance to infection – sip up to a pint twice daily.

- Eat some live yoghurt or other sources of probiotics culture to redress the balance of your bowel bacteria. Insert some (unsweetened) live yoghurt into your vagina to soothe inflammation and destroy thrush infections.

- Candida thrives in an alkaline environment. Mix one part cider vinegar to three parts water as a douche.

- Stress is linked with weakened immunity and thrush. Counteract it with *Yoga*, deep *relaxation* and/or *autohypnosis*.

- Try a *Bach Flower Remedy*, for example Cherry Plum for fear of losing control or Impatiens for irritability and impatience.

- Medical herbalists prescribe compresses and douches using extracts of bramble leaves, comfrey, crab apples, goldenseal and rose petals for vaginal infections.

- Try swabbing your vulva and inner vaginal lips with aloe vera liquid or gel.

- Add two drops of *aromatherapy* essence of juniper, lavender or niauoli to your bathwater, or inhale in steam or from an oil burner.

Drug remedies

o Once the organism causing the infection has been identified, the appropriate antibiotic is prescribed, either as capsules or tablets or in the form of a pessary or cream which you insert into the vagina.

○ Clotrimazole or nystatin pessaries and creams are used to treat thrush, and a large (3 g) single oral dose of amoxicillin treats gonorrhoea.

○ Oral metronidazole is prescribed for *Trichomonas* infection.

SEE YOUR DOCTOR IF...

• Your symptoms remain despite simple home treatments. A swab of your discharge is needed to identify the infective organism and prescribe treatment.

12

Skin, Nail and Hair Ailments

> • Abscesses and boils • Acne • Cold sores (herpes)
> • Corns and calluses • Eczema • Hair loss • Heavy
> perspiration • Hives • Impetigo • Lice • Prickly
> heat and itching • Psoriasis • Ringworm and
> athlete's foot • Sebaceous cysts • Sore, cracked lips
> • Sunburn • Warts and verrucae

▪ Abscesses and Boils

An abscess is a collection of pus in a pocket of healthy tissue. Many start with a puncture wound from, for instance, an insect bite or foreign body which introduces bacteria below the skin. Released toxins activate inflammation and the surrounding tissues thicken, walling off the invaders. The abscess fills with pus, composed of tissue fluid, white blood cells, bacteria (alive and dead) and damaged tissue fragments. Eventually, either the abscess bursts or the surrounding tissues digest and dispose of its contents.

A boil is a small abscess inside a sweat gland or surrounding a hair root. Boils often appear on the back of the neck, within or near the armpits and on the face.

With a skin abscess or boil, you experience pain due to the pus under pressure and the area becomes swollen, red and hot. You may also feel unwell, with aches, pains and other *flu*-like symptoms. Adjacent lymph nodes may also become tender and swollen.

WHAT YOU CAN DO

- Wash and dry sweaty, hairy areas frequently. Add a few drops of antiseptic or of lavender or rosemary oil to bathwater.

- Boost your immunity with a healthy wholefood diet (SEE *Nutritional Medicine*). Drink eight or more glasses of water daily and add some freshly squeezed antioxidant-rich juices – carrot for beta-carotene (provitamin A), citrus fruit for vitamin C and bioflavonoids and pulped bananas for potassium for strong, resilient tissue cells.

- Dab the area with a little tea tree oil as soon as you suspect a boil or abscess may be developing.

- To draw the pus, place a face flannel in boiling water with 2–3 drops of chamomile, clary sage, lavender, sandalwood, southernwood or tea tree essential oil. Wring out and apply to the spot.

- Apply a thick hot poultice of slippery elm powder mixed with runny honey.

- Try these homoeopathic remedies hourly for up to ten doses:

  - To encourage healing after an abscess has been lanced (cut), or for an abscess that refuses to disappear or come to a head: Silicea 6c

- For a chilly and irritable person with a discharging abscess which is very tender and causes sharp shooting pains: Hepar sulph. 6c

- To bring a boil to a head, or for a discharging, very tender boil: Hepar sulph. 6c

- For a weeping but not painful boil: Gunpowder 6c

- Use *acupressure* to boost immunity. Useful points include:

  - Sea of Vitality

  - Three Mile Point

Drug remedies

- Magnesium sulphate paste can be applied below a plaster or small bandage to 'draw' the boil or abscess, i.e. encourage it to develop a head. It will then either burst spontaneously or be ready for lancing to get rid of the pus.

- Antibiotics are prescribed for boils and abscesses.

- NSAIDs (non-steroidal anti-inflammatory drugs) are useful for combating inflammation, throbbing and the generalized aches and pains that sometimes occur.

- Some sufferers may require a paracetamol + codeine combination to control the pain.

SEE YOUR DOCTOR IF...
- Home treatments do not help you.
- You experience recurrent abscess/boil attacks. A general health check is indicated to eliminate diabetes and other causes.
- You need prescription painkillers or antibiotics.

▪ Acne

Acne may be the bane of your life if you're a teenager or (occasionally) somewhat older. The spots typically occur in crops on the face, neck, back and chest in response to the raised testosterone levels that circulate from puberty onwards. This hormone – produced by both sexes but in far larger quantities by boys – boosts the rate of skin cell production and the manufacture of the skin's natural lubricant, sebum.

The (sebaceous) glands that make sebum often become blocked with an oily mixture of dead cells and develop into lumpy red spots or pus-filled pimples. Inevitably boys are more affected than girls, but the skin's condition tends to improve greatly by the late teens or early twenties.

Picking and squeezing spots can be very tempting, but this usually compounds the problem by spreading the bacteria found in and around acne rashes. It can also result in scarring. You're better off keeping your skin scrupulously clean and applying concealer to the worst offenders. Drinking water and freshly squeezed juices and eating fresh fruit and vegetables may also help.

WHAT YOU CAN DO

- Avoid picking or squeezing!

- Wash the affected areas thoroughly twice daily with lukewarm water and a recommended soap or facial wash. Use your hands rather than a flannel (which can harbour skin bacteria). Pat dry with a soft clean towel – never irritate the inflamed spots by scrubbing or rubbing them.

- Drink six to eight glasses of pure water daily (more in hot weather and when you exercise vigorously).

- Aim to eat five portions of raw or lightly cooked fruit and vegetables daily.

- Try cutting down on greasy foods, alcohol, cheese, chocolate, nuts, fizzy drinks and junk food in general. Don't expect results in the first month!

- Some naturopathic doctors recommend drinking 600 ml (1 pint) of mixed carrot, celery and grapefruit juice twice daily.

- Medical herbalists sometimes prescribe mallow flowers and roots, sage flowers, and the leaves of artichoke, burdock and celandine. Try soaking a handful of one or more of these in boiling water for 10 minutes, then straining, cooling and using to bathe acne areas.

- Dab spots with witch hazel neat or mixed with an equal volume of fresh cabbage juice.

- Add 4–5 drops *aromatherapy* essence of lavender to bathwater, or apply it neat to spots. Essences of aspic (old English lavender), calendula, myrrh, myrtle, neroli, patchouli, petitgrain (from orange leaves, twigs and immature fruit) and tea tree are also excellent for acne.

- Avoid unnecessary stress (which aggravates acne). Join a *Yoga* class or buy a *Yoga* or deep *relaxation* tape or video and practise at home several times weekly. Improve poor sleep with a cassette or CD of relaxing sounds to drift off to. The voices of whales or dolphins, a fountain playing, a waterfall trickling over rocks or wind in the trees are all excellent choices.

Drug remedies

○ Anti-bacterial skin preparations (for example benzoyl peroxide solution, metronidazole gel) combat skin infection.

○ Keratolytics (for example benzoyl peroxide, salicylic acid) and abrasives (for example aluminium oxide) peel off superficial skin layers and unblock clogged sebaceous glands.

○ Antibiotic skin products (for example erythromycin, clindamycin) and oral antibiotics (for example minocycline, doxycycline) check unhealthy skin bacteria.

○ Hormones counteract testosterone in female acne sufferers.

○ Retinoid skin and oral products often work best for very severe acne sufferers.

SEE YOUR DOCTOR IF...

• Home treatments fail to help.
• You are becoming depressed about the acne.

▪ Cold Sore (Herpes)

Known medically as Herpes simplex after the virus that causes it, cold sores appear as a cluster of inflamed *blisters* around the mouth or nostrils, often during a *cold* or *sinusitis* attack. Most of us carry the inactive virus all our lives without developing sores, but if you experience one outbreak, you can expect others in the future.

Triggers include a resistance-lowering illness, fever or emotional strain, the premenstrual phase of menstruation (before your period starts) and exposure to strong sunlight or very hot or cold weather. You may feel an itching and tingling before the *blisters* appear, and develop *mouth ulcers* and/or sore red gums. Cold sores irritate and weep before forming a crust, and should not be scratched or picked.

The fluid and crusts are potentially infective, especially to small babies, so handle and kiss these as little as possible during attacks (which last around 7–10 days).

WHAT YOU CAN DO

- Take suitable countermeasures, for example wear a sunblock in bright sunlight.

- Stock up on antioxidants with wholefoods and plenty of fresh fruit and vegetables.

- Try one of these as a daily pick-me-up: pink grapefruit juice flavoured with grated ginger root and 5 ml (1 tsp) runny honey and a handful of fresh mint; or blend equal volumes of tomato juice with freshly squeezed orange juice and add fresh lemon balm or fresh parsley. Serve over ice cubes with a splash of Tabasco or Worcestershire sauce.

- The amino acid lysine may help to ward off cold sores; good sources include fish, chicken, lamb, milk, cheese, beans, brewer's yeast and beansprouts.

- Try cutting down on the amino arginine, found in cereals, seeds, chocolate and peanuts.

- Keep the *blisters* area dry when washing, but moisten with calendula or chamomile lotion (SEE *Herbal Medicine*) two to three times daily to relieve irritation and swelling. Alternatively, use calendula or chamomile essential oil, or lavender or tea tree oil.

- Select an appropriate *Bach Flower Remedy* – possible choices include Agrimony, Aspen, Gorse and Holly.

- Try these homoeopathic remedies four times daily for up to 5 days:
  - When mouth and chin are affected and ulcers form at the corner of the mouth: Rhus tox. 6c

- o For a deep crack in the middle of the lower lip, mouth very dry, sores puffy and burning, pearly *blisters* in lips: Natrum mur. 6c

- o For ulcers inside mouth, gums bleed easily, whole mouth is very sore, especially at night: Sempervivum 6c

- Try these *acupressure* points for boosting your immune defences:

  - o Sea of Consciousness

  - o Three Mile Point

- Counteract tension with deep *relaxation* and *Yoga.*

- Avoid touching eyes and genitals after touching cold sores: Herpes simplex can also cause eye ulceration and genital infection.

Drug remedies

- o Antiseptic soap or face wash for surrounding area.

- o The anti-viral drug aciclovir is available as a cream (SEE ALSO *below*).

SEE YOUR DOCTOR IF...

- Your cold sores last for a fortnight or longer, spread to other areas and/or fail to respond to home measures.
- You also develop fever, severe *mouth ulcers*, sore gums, *headaches* and persistent fatigue.
- Doctors can prescribe anti-viral aciclovir tablets in severe cases and for people such as cancer patients and others with lowered immunity.

▪ Corns and Calluses

Calluses are patches of hard skin on the feet, or occasionally on the hands. They are formed by constant or repeated pressure and you may suffer from them if you wear ill-fitting shoes or high heels or do heavy manual work. Foot deformities such as club foot or bunions and generally going barefoot on hard or rough surfaces can also be responsible. Calluses can be very tender when pressed and diabetic sufferers sometimes develop ulcers underneath them – a complication needing prompt medical attention.

Corns occur on the toes and are also caused by repeated pressure from misshapen feet and unsuitable shoes. Patches of thickened skin get pressed inwards, creating a soft corn between the toes or a hard one elsewhere, with a thick outer coating, surrounding a tiny chalky core or 'seed'.

WHAT YOU CAN DO

- Stop wearing shoes that give rise to callus or corn formation.

- Choose comfortable shoes – open sandals if possible – to allow your feet space to expand fully.

- You can avoid the splaying or shapelessness which many conventional shoe wearers associate with 'sloppy' sandals by buying some with inner moulded surfaces. They encourage your toes to grip, thereby toning the small foot muscles and keeping the foot toned and trim.

- If you have a foot deformity, wear the prescribed shoes. If you dislike their appearance, find out whether you can have their therapeutic aspects incorporated into a shoe with a more pleasing appearance.

- Small defects of the feet can be corrected with orthotics – small plastic inserts that cushion and protect the foot while easing it into the correct anatomical position. Usually these are prescribed by a podiatrist or chiropodist.

- Wash your feet thoroughly with warm soapy water and soak them in the bath whenever you can. Rub calluses gently with pumice stone (available from pharmacies), then dry them thoroughly and apply unscented talcum powder all over your feet and between your toes.

- Try not to cut or poke corns and calluses, especially with an unsterilized blade or needle! It's a job for an expert.

- Massage your feet daily with 15 ml (3 tbsp) plain cooking oil mixed with 10 ml (2 tbsp) glycerine and 3–4 drops of lavender essence. Alternatively, get someone to do it for you. Foot massage is extremely relaxing, sensuous, erotic – and excellent for hard skin of all types!

- Apply herbal calendula (marigold) cream to painful calluses and rub corns with garlic. Fix a slice of garlic over your corns and leave in place overnight.

- See a chiropodist to remove calluses and corns you cannot remove for yourself.

- Try the homoeopathic remedy Antimonium 5c four times daily for up to 2 weeks.

Drug remedies

o Pharmacists sell special plasters to protect painful corns.

o Salicylic acid and lactic acid preparations help to dissolve hard skin when applied to calluses or corns.

> ### SEE YOUR DOCTOR IF...
>
> - You have a foot deformity that is causing painful hard skin conditions of the feet.
> - You are diabetic and suffer from corns, calluses or other foot problems.
> - Home treatments fail to offer relief.

▪ Eczema

Eczema causes dry skin, inflammation and severe irritation. It can also weep, leaving raw red areas which form scabs and become infected.

Atopic eczema is commonest in babies and small children, and tends to occur in families with a history of other allergic (atopic) conditions such as *hayfever, asthma* and *hives* (urticaria). Atopic eczema rash typically appears in skin creases such as the backs of the knees, the front of the elbows and around the neck.

Contact eczema is triggered by an allergy to plants, chemicals or metals, for example poison ivy, tomato leaves, hairdressing products, detergents and nickel jewellery. The hands especially may develop dry, rough, red, itchy patches on the palms and the knuckles.

WHAT YOU CAN DO

- Follow a natural wholefood diet with several daily portions of organic fresh fruit and vegetables. Avoid artificial additives and any dietary items to which you are sensitive.

- Raw juice therapy is often helpful. Try carrot juice 170 ml (7 fl oz) mixed with 140 ml (6 fl oz) each of cucumber and beetroot juice or a mixture of 230 ml (9 fl oz) each of celery and carrot juice.

Nutritionally, juices are best prepared immediately before drinking, but you can compromise by preparing them once daily and keeping them covered in the fridge.

- Supplements of omega-6 and omega-3 essential fatty acids help reduce eczema symptoms. Try 3 × 500 mg capsules EPO (omega-6) twice daily and 1–2 fish oil capsules, or buy the combined product. Try to eat oily fish – tuna, sardines, kippers – once or twice weekly.

- Dab lesions with the contents of one or more EPO capsules.

- Sip chamomile tea and add 4–5 drops of the essential oil to bathwater to calm *anxiety*. Worry and stress aggravate eczema, especially the atopic type.

- Homoeopathic remedies can be useful for severe itching and/or while waiting for professional homoeopathic/medical treatment; take 4 times daily for up to 14 days:

  o For dry burning skin aggravated by cold lotions and creams: Arsenicum 6c

  o For dry and itchy skin and *constipation*: Alumina 6c

  o For dry, rough, red, itchy skin worsened by heat and washing, especially if the sufferer has *diarrhoea* which is worse in the early morning: Sulphur 6c

  o For eczema mainly on the palms and behind the ears, producing a yellow sticky discharge: Graphites 6c

- Learn deep *relaxation* and *Yoga* and practise daily while eczema is present and daily or on alternate days between attacks.

- Try a *Bach Flower Remedy*: Red Chestnut if you are always anticipating misfortune and projecting *anxiety*, Vervain for a stressed nature.

Drug remedies

○ Gammaderm cream containing 20 per cent evening primrose oil is recommended as an emollient (skin softener). When used in atopic eczema, it also aims to rectify, in part, the essential fatty acid deficiency in the skin believed to underlie this form of the complaint.

○ Other emollients can be used, containing, for instance, light liquid and white soft paraffin, zinc oxide, almond oil and/or glycerine.

○ Anti-pruritic (anti-itch) products include the relatively new tacrolimus, which helps to control the allergy symptoms, and pimecrolimus, which has a specifically anti-inflammatory effect on the skin.

○ Antihistamines and steroid creams are also useful, as are antibiotics to control infection.

SEE YOUR DOCTOR IF...

- Simple home treatments do not work.
- Prescribed medications do not work.
- Symptoms worsen or infection develops.

■ Hair Loss

We shed dead hair continually, but if new growth fails to keep pace then the loss becomes apparent. You may have noticed this after having a baby, starting the menopause or during a long illness or interval of nervous strain. Women tend to lose hair from the crown of the head, but male pattern baldness (MPB), which runs in families, involves both a thinning crown and receding hairline, and can lead to complete baldness.

You may lose hair if you suffer from iron deficiency anaemia or an underactive thyroid gland, or if your intake of vitamin A or selenium is too high.

Alopecia (loss of hair) is a recognized side-effect of some anti-cancer drugs, anti-coagulant therapy, some antibiotics, steroids, anti-convulsants and oral contraceptives. Alopecia can also result from B vitamin deficiency, particularly of biotin and inositol. Providing the cause of your alopecia can be treated, your hair should regrow, but hair follicles destroyed by ageing, MPB and scalp diseases like *ringworm* cannot produce any further hair.

WHAT YOU CAN DO

- Follow a wholefood diet, making sure that you take in sufficient protein, vitamins and minerals, many of which contribute to healthy hair and skin. The essential amino acids provided by first-class protein are needed to promote hair growth and healthy skin. Liver, wheatgerm, pulses and beans, tofu, low-fat cheese and milk, lean meat, poultry and fish are excellent choices.

- Good sources of inositol (a vitamin-like nutrient involved in lipid metabolism) include cantaloupe melon, grapefruit, cabbage, peanuts and raisins; biotin, a B vitamin which helps to prevent baldness and hair greying, is found in egg yolk, milk, nuts, fruit and wholegrain rice. Alternatively, take a vitamin B supplement for 2–3 months.

- If you are anaemic, top up your iron with lean red meat, asparagus, beans, oatmeal, kidney and liver. You'll find zinc in steak, lamb, lean pork, wheatgerm, pumpkin seeds, eggs and ground mustard.

- Sip 300 ml (½ pint) of freshly squeezed lettuce juice daily. You can improve the slightly insipid flavour by adding a handful of watercress, parsley or mint. This is not claimed to increase hair growth, but it provides a useful spectrum of vitamins and minerals, and has a calming effect upon frayed nerves.

- Many shampoos and hair preparations claim to boost hair growth. Evening primrose oil, tea tree oil, aloe vera extract, jojoba and pantothenic acid (one of the B vitamins) are all likely to help. Evening primrose oil is also beneficial to skin, hair and nails. Take 2–3 (500 mg) capsules daily for several months to improve hair condition.

- Take a herbal remedy containing horsetail, a source of the nutrient silica, which is essential to hair health.

- Take some supplementary kelp, too, which is rich in iodine, for a healthy thyroid gland.

- If nervous tension has contributed to your hair loss, practise *relaxation* and *Yoga* daily.

- Try Indian head massage – a wonderfully soothing, energizing and stimulating holistic practice which benefits scalp health and overall tranquillity.

Drug remedies

- There is no cure for alopecia other than treatment, where possible, of the underlying cause.

- The drug finasteride, prescribed for men with non-cancerous enlargement of the prostate gland, sometimes helps to delay hair loss in MPB.

SEE YOUR DOCTOR IF...

- You experience unexplained hair loss.

■ Heavy Perspiration

This can be an embarrassing problem and worrying about it is likely to worsen matters. Naturopathic practitioners believe that excessive perspiration happens because we need to excrete surplus waste matter, and it should not, therefore, be hampered by the use of an antiperspirant. You could follow these tips and actively suppress perspiration only if necessary.

Apart from obvious causes such as heavy manual work, aerobic exercise, hot weather and central heating, sweating heavily can result from bingeing on alcohol. Hot spicy foods also raise the body temperature. Wearing nylon and other man-made fibres concentrates body heat and encourages perspiration.

Vitamin B1 deficiency can be responsible and both the *menopause* and *anxiety* are familiar causes. You can also sweat profusely if you have a fever, are severely overweight or suffer from hypoglycaemia (low blood sugar) (SEE *Blood Sugar Imbalance*), an overactive thyroid gland and rarer conditions such as Hodgkin's disease (which is similar to leukaemia) and tuberculosis.

WHAT YOU CAN DO

- Shed surplus weight.

- Exercise outdoors when it is cool or inside in an air-conditioned gym.

- Put aside all tightly fitting belts, underclothes, trousers, shoes, etc. You are better off with a handful of cool comfortable cotton bras, pants, shirts, etc. and loose-fitting skirts, nightdresses, tops and trousers also in cotton and natural fibres that allow the skin to breathe. Change clothes daily.

- Shower night and morning to remove all sweat and odour (which comes from bacteria that breed in sweat).

- Avoid highly spiced foods, strong tea and coffee, and opt for cooling salads, still or sparkling mineral water or freshly squeezed fruit and vegetable juices. Try a mixture of carrot, cucumber and apple, or blend a pulped banana with orange juice to replace some of the potassium you lose in sweat.

- Sip cooling rosehip, lime-flower or chamomile tea. Try it iced in summer, with a slice of lime or lemon.

- Limit yourself to a maximum of 2–3 units of alcohol at any one time.

- Bathe your forehead, underarms, pubic area and perineum (between your legs) with cool water to which you have added a few drops of tea tree or lavender oil. Take great care that none of this solution enters your body.

- Try these homoeopathic remedies 4 times daily for up to 2 weeks:

  o For a slim cold-feeling individual with sweaty offensive-smelling feet: Silicea 6c

  o For someone who gets hot and sweaty on the forehead and scalp, and has early morning *diarrhoea*: Sulphur 6c

  o For someone with strong and sickly-smelling sweat, aggravated by extremes of temperature: Mercurius 6c

  o For an overweight person who is chilly and clammy, with sour-smelling sweat and sweating of the head region, especially at night: Calcarea 6c

  o For someone with offensive perspiration, especially under the arms and on the feet, whose right foot may be hot and left foot chilly: Lycopodium 6c

Drug remedies

○ Pharmaceutical antiperspirants, for example Anhydrol, Driclor, containing aluminium chloride hexahydrate.

○ Pharmaceutical dusting powder Zeasorb containing chloroxylenol, aluminium dihydroxyallantoinate and cellulose.

SEE YOUR DOCTOR IF...

- You have unexplained weight loss – your thyroid gland could be overactive.
- For a blood sugar check, if simple dietary measures against hypoglycaemia do not help.
- If you are distressed by your perspiration pattern despite home treatments. Occasionally, an operation on abdominal nerve fibres controlling perspiration is possible.

▪ Hives

Also known as urticaria or nettle-rash, hives is a rash of raised lumps or weals, often whitish in colour and surrounded by red skin. It resembles nettle stings, is intensely itchy and is usually brought on by contact with an allergen. This may be a food or drug to which you know you are sensitive, or something you have come across before, without apparent harm. Common triggers include penicillin and other antibiotics, food additives, foods such as fish, shellfish, strawberries or eggs, insect bites and stings, and the ingredients of a perfume, soap or cosmetic.

Heat, cold and sunlight can all raise weals in sensitive people. Importantly, severe stress and *anxiety* can irritate the condition, and even trigger an attack when no apparent allergen can be identified. You stand an increased risk of hives if you suffer from other so-called atopic complaints such as *eczema, asthma* or *hayfever*.

WHAT YOU CAN DO

- Avoid known personal triggers.

- Have a wholefood diet without processed foods.

- Recommended juices for *asthma* which can also relieve urticaria include carrot with a little spinach, carrot and celery (any proportions), and grapefruit.

- Take a cold shower and/or apply an ice pack (which can be a covered pack of frozen peas, for example) to patches of the rash.

- Apply calamine lotion, which soothes and cools the intense itch. Keep the lotion in the fridge between applications.

- Hold a fresh cabbage leaf against the hives rash or bathe it with some freshly squeezed cabbage juice.

- Meet fire with fire! Unless you are allergic to stinging nettles, pick the new tops of plants in the spring or autumn, wearing gloves, squeeze out the juice and mix with unperfumed cold cream. Apply to the rash twice daily.

- If stress brings you out in hives (*anxiety* and grief are known triggers), practise deep *relaxation, Yoga* and/or meditation, or seek some counselling to help you deal with your problems.

- Try *Bach Flower Remedies* Sweet Chestnut for intolerable grief, Agrimony for internalized anxiety or Star of Bethlehem for grief, distress and to help you recover from a fright or shock.

- These homoeopathic remedies can help:
  - Use Apis 30c every minute until help arrives, for swelling of lips, throat and tongue.

o For a rash caused by stinging nettles or some other plant, aggravated by contact with water, scratching or touching, give hourly for up to ten doses, during an attack or while awaiting medical attention: Urtica 6c

Drug remedies

o Antihistamines in tablet form, for example hydroxyzine, chlorpheniramine or desloratadine would be prescribed.

o An antihistamine injection may be required for severe hives. It would also be used as an emergency measure in a full-blown allergy attack which can occasionally develop when hives appear. Symptoms include a swollen tongue, eyes and lips. The throat can swell dramatically and cut off the air supply. (SEE ALSO *homoeopathic remedies above.*)

SEE YOUR DOCTOR IF...

- *Urgently* if you develop the swelling and breathing difficulty described above.
- Home treatments have no effect.
- You suffer repeated attacks.
- You need help identifying your personal trigger(s). Tests can be carried out to identify certain allergens and a course of desensitizing injections given to overcome the problem.

▪ Impetigo

Also known as 'school sores', impetigo is caused by streptococcal or staphylococcal bacteria invading the skin's outer layer, the epidermis. Tiny *blisters* appear in patches anywhere on the body, but most often around the nose and the mouth, arms and legs. You will notice a stinging and tingling in the affected area before the *blisters* burst, forming crusty scabs like brown sugar. The lesions, which can be very itchy, weep and ooze yellow fluid and pus, which can then irritate and further infect the surrounding skin.

You pass on the infection by picking or touching the *blisters*, then touching another part of the body (or another person). The bacteria are also spread by sharing towels, face flannels, handkerchiefs, drinking mugs and dummies. The condition usually clears up with antibiotic treatment, but it can have serious consequences such as kidney infection in newborn babies and chronically sick or convalescent children.

WHAT YOU CAN DO

- Always wash your hands thoroughly after touching the affected area.

- Keep towels and flannels away from those of other family members.

- Keep your child away from school and let the school know the cause (or see your GP, as below).

- Bathe the impetigo lesions with dilute TCP several times daily (follow the instructions on the bottle).

- Alternatively, add 4–5 drops of benzoin, chamomile, patchouli or tea tree essential oil to a basin of warm water and bathe as above.

- Cider vinegar enthusiasts claim beneficial results from dabbing impetigo lesions up to a dozen times a day with a clean pad or tissue (each time) dipped in this vinegar.

- Try propolis, a natural antibacterial substance manufactured by bees to maintain infection-free hives. Apply the ointment several times daily after bathing and drying as recommended above.

- Calendula *aromatherapy* oil combats impetigo skin lesions. Add 4–5 drops to 10 ml (2 tsp) wheatgerm oil and apply once a day. Make up fresh each time.

- Homoeopathic remedies to relieve impetigo symptoms – use hourly for up to ten doses:

  o When the impetigo is accompanied by feeling chilly and mentally restless, but at the same time physically exhausted: Arsenicum 6c

  o For *blisters* around the mouth and nostrils, especially in children: Antimonium 6c

  o For *blisters* – particularly on the scalp – which form thick scabs and ooze pus that irritates the adjoining skin: Mezereum 6c

  o For inflamed, oozing *blisters* which are worst on the testicles: Croton 6c

- Help your immune defence system to overcome this infection. Discard fatty, sugary convenience foods with their chemical additives, eat fresh fruit and vegetables at least twice daily and try these juices, recommended for septic spots and skin eruptions: pure grape juice, 250 ml (½ pint) four times daily, or the same quantity of carrot and cucumber (in 2:1 proportions) with some fresh garlic and a handful of fresh spinach added.

Drug remedies

o Antiseptic powders and creams containing povidone-iodine, cetrimide, chlorhexidine, hydrogen peroxide, triclosan and/or benzalkonium chloride.

○ Antibiotic/antibacterial creams and ointments such as mupirocin, fusidic acid and polymyxin B.

○ Antibiotics such as flucloxacillin to be taken by mouth.

SEE YOUR DOCTOR IF...

• Your child develops impetigo.
• For all but the most trivial sores, because an antibiotic course will be needed.
• Home treatments do not help.

▪ Lice

Head lice are parasites that live on the scalp. They suck blood, lay tiny white eggs ('nits') on the hair and cause intense itching. Some people feel embarrassed and indignant if their child is affected, but in fact lice prefer clean, frequently washed hair.

Head lice pass like wildfire, especially in schools; if one family member is affected you will need to treat the whole family. Males suffer less often than females because their hormones offer them some protection.

Pubic lice ('crabs') are a crab-shaped species infesting hair in the pubic, anal and perineal areas (between the legs). The itching they cause is especially severe at night, and they are passed on by sexual intercourse and infested bedclothes. Lice eggs take 12–14 days to hatch, and you may not notice pubic lice symptoms for up to a fortnight after contact. Scratching damages the skin and can lead to bacterial infection. Nearby lymph glands become tender and swollen, and you may need an antibiotic.

WHAT YOU CAN DO

- Treat yourself with one of the medications listed on page 242.

Head lice

- For head lice, burn all head gear and alert the school doctor or nurse if applicable.

- Remove all comfort blankets (offer a 'safe' temporary replacement!), soft toys and similar objects, and store in a tightly fastened bin liner for three weeks. The lice cannot live without a human host and after 3 weeks any newly hatched lice will be dead.

- Wash brushes and combs, bedding, clothing, cushion and upholstery covers that could harbour lice or nits.

- You can sometimes pick nits out of the hair by hand or with a fine-toothed comb moistened with Listerine mouthwash or white vinegar.

- Use tea tree oil shampoo to help prevent head lice. Allow hair to dry naturally (hair driers interfere with many anti-lice treatments).

- Treat head lice with about 20 ml (4 tsp) vodka mixed with 12 drops geranium essence. Rub into scalp at night and wash off in the morning.

Pubic lice

- Shave or cut hair very short in the pubic, perineal and anal areas, also any beard or moustache.

- Wash bedding and clothing.

- For repeated infestations, it may help to get your mattress professionally cleaned.

- Bath often and wear clean underwear daily.

- Add *aromatherapy* essence of cedarwood, southernwood or tea tree to bathwater. Bathe and soak affected areas twice daily.

- Try *acupressure* for troublesome itching, whatever the cause. Use Crooked Pond.

Drug remedies

o Benzyl benzoate emulsion combats head lice and crabs.

o Malathion liquid acts similarly.

o Phenothrin lotion is highly effective against head and pubic lice and their eggs.

o Carbaryl lotion will get rid of head lice.

o Permethrin lotion is active against crab lice and their eggs.

o For frequent infestations, you need to alternate the products to prevent the lice from becoming resistant. And always check the suitability of a product for children. You can get all head lice preparations apart from carbaryl without a prescription.

SEE YOUR DOCTOR IF...

- Home treatment methods have not helped.
- You need advice on avoiding further infestation.
- Any of the scratch sites become infected.

▪ Prickly Heat and Itching

You are most likely to suffer from prickly heat if you are fair-skinned, visit the tropics or sub-tropics, and fail to keep cool. Like other sufferers, you may find the sensation of 'thousands of minute needles prickling the skin' almost unbearable.

Overworked sweat glands blocked by sebum are the underlying cause. In hot wet conditions these glands produce extra sweat, swell because their openings are blocked and form *blisters.* These burst (creating the unique prickling sensation) and the skin becomes inflamed. Triggers include damp heat, clothing, being overweight, using soap too often and producing too much sebum.

Other familiar sources of itching include *piles,* jaundice, *eczema, psoriasis, hives, ringworm,* head *lice,* scabies and *insect bites and stings.*

WHAT YOU CAN DO

Prickly heat

- Stay cool! Avoid hot showers and baths, hot drinks and spicy foods. Wear cool loose-fitting cotton clothing and go naked when you can.

- Use soap once daily only – washing too much sebum from the skin stimulates it to produce more.

- Lose excess weight – it makes you sweat more, and the sweat gathers between rolls of flesh, aggravating the problem.

- Homoeopathic remedies:

  o Apis 30c 2-hourly for up to ten doses – you can repeat this daily if necessary

  o As a preventative, use Sol 30c once daily during exposure for up to 3 weeks in every 4.

- Mosquito, flea and other insect bites itch because the skin cells release histamine in response. Dab bites with TCP, tea tree or lavender oil, or use any of these to make an ice-cold compress (refresh as needed).

Fleas

- Fleas need to be eradicated – launder clothing and pets' beds, powder/spray and vacuum carpets and upholstery, and treat pets with a specially formulated anti-flea product. Cats and dogs can also be rendered flea-free with a daily garlic or garlic-and-fenugreek tablet (give two during hot weather). Flea collars work well, too.

Mosquitoes

- Mosquitoes and similar insects also hate garlic. Eat two to three fresh cloves every day, take garlic tablets or capsules, or try a supplement of the B vitamin biotin, which also produces an unpleasant aroma detectable to insects.

Scabies

- Scabies is due to a parasite (mite) which burrows below the skin to lay eggs, which then hatch. Intensely itchy red lumps appear on hands, wrists, genitals or elsewhere, and the creatures' characteristic tracks may be seen as raised white burrows below the skin. You pick up scabies by personal and sexual contact or from infested clothing or bedding, especially in overcrowded, unhygienic surroundings.

- Launder all clothing and bedding and apply lavender or tea tree oil to the rash.

- Homoeopathic remedy: all family members should take 1 × Sulphur 30c tablet every 12 hours for up to 3 days, whether affected or not, provided they do not suffer from *eczema*.

Drug remedies

○ Hydroxyzine and other antihistamine medication (SEE *Hives*).

○ Emollient lotion, cream and bath oil containing oatmeal extract.

○ A pharmaceutical emollient cream with chamomile extract.

○ Anti-itch (and anti-scabies) cream with crotamiton.

○ For scabies rashes, malathion liquid or benzyl benzoate emulsion, used according to packet directions.

SEE YOUR DOCTOR IF...

● Home treatments do not help.
● Rashes or bites become infected.

■ Psoriasis

A psoriasis rash can take many forms, but typically it consists of red raised patches shedding silvery flakes of dead skin. The faulty mechanism is the over-rapid production of new cells in the skin's outer layer (epidermis). Keratin (a tough, fibrous protein normally protecting skin, nails and hair) cannot be formed quickly enough, and unsightly patches can develop on your knees, elbows, scalp and the sacral area at the base of the spine. Affected nails become thick, discoloured and rough, and can come detached from their nail bed and fall off.

Psoriasis is neither contagious nor invariably itchy or sore, and most sufferers agree that its worst aspect is its appearance. It is a chronic (ongoing) condition, commonly found between the ages of 15 and 30, and it flares up in response to stress, *anxiety*, streptococcal (and other) infections and the use of chloroquine, a drug prescribed for *arthritis* and malaria. You may also develop psoriasis-related *arthritis* in your fingers, knees, feet and ankles.

WHAT YOU CAN DO

- Essential fatty acids are beneficial for psoriasis. Eat a wholefood diet with oily fish as a protein meal several times a week, or take a daily fish oil supplement. Eat five or more portions of fresh organic fruit and veg daily, drink six to eight glasses of water (minimum) and try this juice: apple and carrot mixed (at least one third of one to two thirds of the other, or equal volumes of the two). Aim to drink 500–600 ml (20–24 fl oz) daily.

- Top up your essential nutrient levels with a multivitamin/mineral supplement and add some zinc and some vitamin B complex to encourage healthy skin growth and to help counteract the effects of stress.

- Medical herbalists may prescribe preparations of chamomile, lavender, sage, thyme or lime flowers. Lime-flower tea is especially soothing to frayed nerves.

- You can swab itchy, angry psoriasis patches with witch hazel solution and apply calendula cream to soften the scaly crust and soothe the inflammation.

- *Aromatherapy* essence of cajeput is said to be useful for psoriasis. Add 5–6 drops to bathwater or 3–4 drops to 20 ml (4 tsp) of almond oil and massage gently into your rash.

- Practise *relaxation* or *Yoga* regularly. Tension and emotional turmoil are known to be directly linked to flare-ups of psoriasis.

- Try a gentle *Bach Flower Remedy* – those for *eczema* may help.

- Homoeopathic remedies to be taken four times daily for up to 14 days:

  ○ For psoriasis which is worse in winter and aggravated by the cold: Petroleum 6c

○ For an extremely scaly psoriasis rash, irritated by warmth: Kali ars. 6c

○ For dry red itchy patches worsened by baths, especially if the sufferer often feels too hot: Sulphur 30c

○ When skin behind the ears is affected and producing yellow pus: Graphites 6c

Drug remedies

○ Dithranol and related products aim at reversing the faulty cellular mechanism underlying psoriasis.

○ Coal tar products can prove very useful – a coal tar shampoo containing coconut oil and salicylic acid helps beat psoriasis of the scalp.

○ Steroid creams and ointments reduce the inflammation and other symptoms.

○ Other measures exist for severe and resistant psoriasis.

SEE YOUR DOCTOR IF...

- Simple home measures do not help symptoms.
- Infection or other troublesome symptoms develop.

▪ Ringworm and Athlete's Foot

Ringworm, a very common skin infection, is caused by the fungus Tinea. You may have found a crimson ring-shaped patch somewhere on your body, possibly in a dark moist place between covered folds of skin. The centre heals before the periphery, hence the shape, and the inflammation is caused by irritation from the fungus's waste products.

Tinea also infects the scalp, causing scaly patches and *hair loss*; the groin, where it is called jock-itch; the hands, trunk, face and beard, and the nails. Infected nails crumble, become misshapen, separate from the underlying nail bed and eventually drop off.

The same fungus is responsible for athlete's foot, which can cause the most punishing itch if you are obliged to wear socks and lace-up shoes or boots. The infected skin reddens, then dies, coming away in large white moist flakes.

WHAT YOU CAN DO

- Continue treatments for 2–3 weeks after the infection has cleared, to destroy all fungal spores.

- Boost your immunity with a wholefood high-raw diet.

- Fresh oranges, grapefruit and other citrus fruit supply vitamin C and bioflavonoids, found in the membranes and pith. Make lemon- or limeade using the flesh and large curls of the thickly peeled washed skin.

- Carrot juice supplies beta-carotene (provitamin A) and fish, milk and cheese supply vitamin D, both vital to the skin's health. Choose low-fat dairy products and oily fish such as tuna, sardines and kippers.

- Wheatbran, wheatgerm, liver, kidney, heart cantaloupe melon, blackstrap molasses, cabbage, milk, eggs and beef are excellent sources of many of the B vitamins needed by a healthy immune system and to counterbalance stress.

- Vitamin E accelerates skin healing. You will find this in cold-pressed vegetable oils, broccoli, Brussels sprouts, leafy green vegetables, especially spinach, vitamin-enriched flour and cereals, wholegrain cereals and eggs. You can also buy vitamin E capsules and tablets and apply the oil from a capsule (or sold separately) to the lesions twice daily.

- Mix a little bicarbonate of soda with water to make a paste, apply it gently to the lesions, leave in place for 5 minutes then rinse clean and dry.

- Dab the lesions with cider vinegar, then drink some to boost immunity! Take 30 ml (2 tbsp) of the vinegar, dilute with a little water if you wish, add a heaped teaspoon of organic honey and a few fresh sage leaves or a pinch of the dried herb, if liked.

- Propolis ointment often works well for Tinea infections.

- Dissolve 40 ml (8 tsp) ordinary salt in 1,200 ml (2 pints) of warm water and soak your feet in the solution for 10 minutes daily until your athlete's foot has cleared. Add 4–5 drops of *aromatherapy* essence of clary sage, pine or tea tree for extra benefit.

- Freshen smelly shoes each night with a good spray of Febreze, or shake sodium bicarbonate (cooking soda) into your shoes and empty them out each morning.

Drug remedies

○ Anti-fungal creams such as sulconazole, econazole; amorolfine nail lacquer.

○ Nystatin plus chlorhexidine – an anti-fungal/antiseptic combination for fungal skin infections alone or together with bacterial skin infection.

○ Doctors can also prescribe terbinafine or griseofulvin tablets.

SEE YOUR DOCTOR IF...

• Self-treatment does not help.

▪ Sebaceous Cyst

You may have found a smooth round whitish swelling on your scalp or neck and been told by your doctor that it was a sebaceous cyst. This non-cancerous harmless growth develops when the opening of a sebaceous gland becomes clogged – the production of the skin lubricant, sebum, inside the gland, continues for a time, forcing the gland to enlarge.

Occasionally, sebaceous cysts disappear. Usually they remain the same size for years, causing no problems unless they become infected (apart from their appearance, their rubbing on collars and their getting in the way when you comb your hair). Rarely, such cysts just go on growing, forming a huge, solid swelling or 'wen' several inches across on the head or neck.

When infected, the bacteria multiply within, producing pus. The build-up of pressure can cause the cyst to burst, discharging a mixture of semi-liquid solid pus and semi-solid sebum. You may want to have an enlarging cyst removed in a small operation performed under local anaesthetic, depending upon the success of self-help measures.

WHAT YOU CAN DO

• Eat for a healthy skin! Avoid junk and processed foods and saturated animal fat, and follow a wholefood diet rich in omega-6 and omega-3 essential fatty acids (found respectively in cold-pressed vegetable oils and evening primrose oil supplements and in oily fish, for example herring, mackerel, sardines, tuna, and in fish oil supplements).

- Eat five or more portions of fresh fruit and vegetables daily, drink at least six to eight glasses of water daily, and try this beta-carotene and vitamin C-rich juice: carrot and tomato, mixed in equal proportions, served if you like over ice cubes with sprigs of fresh parsley and/or garden mint. You can juice the carrots yourself, but home-juiced tomatoes tend to disappoint. Instead, use a packet or bottled variety by a dependable brand. Aim to drink 500–600 ml (20–24 fl oz) daily.

- Top up your essential nutrient levels with a multivitamin/mineral supplement and add some zinc and vitamin B complex to encourage healthy skin growth.

- Discourage sebum production by resisting the urge to wash your neck and scalp too frequently. Once or twice daily is ample – and dab any greasy-looking areas daily after washing with neat aspic, benzoin or tea tree aromatherapy essence.

- Try these homoeopathic remedies for a troublesome or infected cyst – a dose every 8 hours for up to 5 days:

  ○ For a cyst producing pus: Hepar sulph. 30c

  ○ For a cyst on the scalp which is sensitive to the touch and whose skin covering is flaking: Baryta 30c

Drug remedies

○ There are no drug remedies for sebaceous cysts, but you can help to prevent them by treating high sebum-producing areas with an anti-bacterial/anti-fungal shampoo such as Cleanel, containing (among other ingredients) cetrimide and undecenoic acid, or a scalp ointment such as Cocois, containing sulphur, salicylic acid and coal tar in coconut oil.

SEE YOUR DOCTOR IF...

- You develop any lump anywhere on your body – sebaceous cysts are harmless but they do need to be identified to eliminate other causes.
- You have a sebaceous cyst and would like it removed.
- Your sebaceous cyst steadily increases in size.
- Your cyst starts to 'point' or bursts and discharges its contents. You may require a course of antibiotics.

▪ Sore, Cracked Lips

Sore, cracked lips are a common problem, particularly in the winter when cold winds cause chapping. You may be prone to them if you have a dry skin, you spend a lot of time out of doors or you fail to dry your lips after washing, eating or drinking. The small cracks sting and can bleed, while the dry, rough flakes of dead skin (its outer layer) irritate and catch on clothing.

It's tempting to pick at them and peel the skin off, but this only aggravates the soreness. Other causes of cracked lips include dehydration, especially during a fever, and (occasionally) long-term poor nutrition.

WHAT YOU CAN DO

- Dry your lips thoroughly whenever moist and avoid licking them when nervous or upset.
- Use a lip salve or Vaseline when outside in the cold or indoors in a dry atmosphere.

- Choose a rich creamy lipstick containing a moisturizer rather than the matt type which can dry lips further. Stick to lip salve rather than a cosmetic when your lips are dry and sore.

- Do not peel dead skin fragments – instead apply a mild antiseptic cream several times daily.

- Keep well hydrated with eight or more glasses of water a day, and more if you are running a temperature.

- Babies and toddlers often suffer from chapping below and around the mouth, due to dribbling or drops of spilt drink. Keep this skin area clean and debris-free and dry it after wiping with a wet flannel, particularly in cold windy weather. Antiseptic cream is generally sufficient to relieve the inflammation and soreness.

- If you are counting calories and/or cutting down on fat, remember to include some plant and fish oils regularly. Both omega-6 and omega-3 polyunsaturates (SEE *Nutritional Medicine*) are vital for healthy, lubricated skin, as are many of the nutrients supplied by raw or lightly cooked fruit and vegetables.

- Evening primrose oil, rich in omega-6 GLA (gamma-linolenic acid), relieves skin dryness. Take 1,000–2,000 mg daily (alone or combined with fish oil) for cracked lips and chapping. You can also soften a capsule in a little warm water and squeeze out the contents to apply directly to your lips.

- Vitamin E also works well, taken as a supplement or applied as oil to the dry area.

- Silica helps to strengthen the skin and is found in the herb horsetail.

- One traditional remedy recommends moisturizing chapped lips (or other areas) with steam or warm water, then sealing with a thin coating of vegetable shortening or unsalted butter. You then wait for 20 minutes, remove excess grease with a tissue and take a warm bath or shower.

Drug remedies

○ Emollients – creams and salves based on lanolin, light liquid and soft paraffin, chamomile extract and/or almond oil help to restore oils and moisture to chapped lips and combat irritation. Apply two to three times daily or as needed.

○ Antiseptic creams – with chlorhexidine or cetrimide help to guard against infection. Combined with liquid paraffin, they also soothe and promote rapid healing. Apply two to three times daily.

○ Multivitamin supplements may be prescribed on the NHS, if you are recovering from a debilitating illness, for example, or have problems with fat absorption.

SEE YOUR DOCTOR IF...

● You develop infected lip cracks despite antiseptic creams, or for persistent, irritating chapping.

▪ Sunburn

We've nearly all been caught by the sun at some time. You may try to avoid it on hot cloudless days if you are very fair-skinned because of the link with skin cancer, but it's still possible to get burned in unexpected places. Sunscreen provides protection to face, arms and legs, but the tops of the feet, for instance, can suffer severe burns from the hot sun when you wear open sandals, as can your window-side upper arm and elbow when you are driving.

You will first notice patches of red, very tender skin which later form *blisters* containing a straw-coloured liquid. The larger and more numerous the *blisters*, the more your body has been depleted of vital tissue fluid. If the *blisters* are popped with an unsterilized needle, infection can set in.

Sunburn pain can be excruciating and, combined with the generalized effects of too much exposure to the sun, can give you a *headache* and nausea, too.

WHAT YOU CAN DO

- Wear a sunscreen with an adequate UV protective factor.

- On holiday/the beach, phase sunbathing so that your skin can produce more melanin, the pigmented protective barrier dark-skinned people have. Start with 15 minutes the first day and increase this by 15 minutes daily – or by 15 minutes every second or third day if you are pale-skinned.

- For burned areas, remove rings, bracelets and other jewellery (swelling may occur later), then immerse the burned skin in cold water for 10–15 minutes.

- Leave *blisters* to form. They will disappear or can be treated medically, if necessary, when you are feeling better.

- Apply aloe vera liquid or gel. Clinical trials have shown it to be a powerful soothing anti-infective treatment for burns, promoting early healing.

- Apply neat lavender essential oil to burned areas, or make a cold compress, adding 6–7 drops of oil to a small basin of iced water. Use to saturate a piece of clean muslin or cotton, wring the cloth out and apply it to the area. Moisten and reapply as often as you need to. You can make similar cold compresses using benzoin, clary sage, eucalyptus, geranium, patchouli or tea tree.

- Sip chamomile tea, adding a slice or two of fresh ginger root. Your nerves will be soothed and the ginger will combat any nausea due to sun exposure. Alternatively, make a spritzer from a glass of ginger wine and sparkling mineral water, or opt for some iced non-alcoholic ginger beer.

- Take a painkiller to relieve sunburn pain and *headache*. The NSAIDs (non-steroidal anti-inflammatory drugs) such as naproxen and ibuprofen relieve pain and counteract inflammation; paracetamol + codeine combinations are also effective.

Drug remedies

○ Sunscreens with an efficiently high UV protective factor.

○ Antiseptic emollients such as Sudocrem containing lanolin, zinc oxide, benzyl benzoate (among other ingredients), calamine preparations and creams containing crotamiton, for example Eurax.

○ NSAIDs or paracetamol+codeine combinations can help to quell the burning pain.

○ Other emollients containing, for instance, light liquid and white soft paraffin; zinc oxide, almond oil and/or glycerine.

○ Antibiotic creams or tablets to take by mouth may be prescribed to offer protection against or treat infection.

SEE YOUR DOCTOR IF...

- Your sunburn is extensive and/or is unrelieved by home measures.
- Popped blisters weep and might become infected.

- You feel ill and nauseous from sunburn pain and over-exposure.

■ Warts and Verrucae

The chances are that you have had a wart or verruca at some time. Both types of wart are small, tough, non-cancerous growths in the outer layer of the skin, developing on the fingers, feet and elsewhere. Warts on the hands look unsightly and can bleed if you accidentally catch them, but they rarely hurt. Foot warts – verrucae – which have your body weight pressing them into your flesh, are usually painful. There's often little to see of a verruca, other than a tender swelling on the sole of your foot with a small dark centre.

Warts and verrucae are caused by a highly contagious virus. Warts on the upper body, hands, etc. often multiply into large clusters and you can pass them on by contact with an open cut or scratch. Verrucae can be caught from swimming pools, gyms and other areas where people habitually go barefoot.

WHAT YOU CAN DO

- Eat a wholefood diet and take regular exercise to boost your immune defences. Foods rich in antioxidants are excellent choices, especially fresh fruit and vegetables with a high content of beta-carotene (provitamin A), vitamin C with bioflavonoids and vitamin E. Green tea is extremely rich in antioxidants, too, and you could start by substituting one cup of it per day for Indian tea or coffee.

- Take care not to spread warts or verrucae – keep your hands to yourself while waiting for treatments to work! Cover verrucae with a waterproof plaster when using changing rooms and similar facilities. Wash your socks regularly and do not pick, poke at or cut warts, wherever they happen to be.

- Tea tree oil is active against wart-causing viruses. Apply it neat or in a cream twice daily to every warty lesion, then leave them alone to obtain full benefit.

- Tincture of thuja, derived from a variety of cedar found in the USA, Canada and the Orient, is another potent wart treatment. However, it is potentially toxic and best used under expert professional guidance.

- Try these homoeopathic remedies every 12 hours for up to 12 weeks:

  ○ For soft, fleshy, cauliflower-like warts, especially on the back of the head, which ooze and bleed easily: Thuja 6c

  ○ For warts on the hands: Kali mur. 6c

  ○ For warts on the palms which tend to be sweaty: Natrum mur. 6c

  ○ You can also apply thuja mother tincture (SEE *Homoeopathy*) to the warts twice daily and cover them with a plaster.

- Medical herbalists recommend applying celandine juice on a slice of fresh garlic directly to the wart and protecting the surrounding area with a plaster or a little Vaseline. You can also use dandelion sap – the milky juice that appears from freshly cut dandelion stems – best applied directly from the stem. Protect surrounding skin from its corrosive action as above.

- Acupuncture boosts the immune defence system – you may find this useful in getting rid of warts.

Drug remedies

o Anti-wart ointments, gels, etc. containing formaldehyde, salicylic acid, silver nitrate or glutaraldehyde break warts down after they have been applied daily for several weeks.

o Podophyllin ointment acts more quickly by attacking the wart virus-infected cells.

SEE YOUR DOCTOR IF...

- You need confirmation that a lesion is a wart or verruca.
- You would like your warts medically removed, normally by freezing.

13

Nervous System Ailments

---

* Anxiety * Carpal tunnel syndrome * Depression
* Dizzy spells * Headaches and migraine
* ME (myalgic encephalomyelitis) * Memory
problems * Sciatica * Shingles * Tinnitus

▪ Anxiety

All of us feel anxious at times, particularly when faced with stress
we are unable to control. We learn to deal with it for the most part
through reasoning strategies, using diversions to take our minds
off our problems, and simply from the learned experience that
most of the things that worry us are eventually resolved. However,
anxiety becomes a medical problem when it starts to control *us*
and interferes with our happiness, relationships and health.

Free-floating anxiety is hard to bear because you experience
anxiety without knowing why. The physical symptoms include a
dry mouth, racing heartbeat, stomach pain, a frequent need to

open the bladder or bowels, increased or decreased appetite and disturbed sleep.

Cognitive symptoms include memory lapses, losing things, losing the thread of what others are saying, poor concentration and a reduced ability to make decisions and complete everyday tasks. Emotionally, you may feel low, with a tendency to *depression* and a feeling of dread on facing each day.

WHAT YOU CAN DO

- Prevent an anxiety build-up by discussing your concerns with a friend, partner or colleague. Make a Plan A and an alternative Plan B for dealing with each of your problems. Revise the list regularly in the light of new developments.

- Aerobic exercise is an excellent anxiety antidote – if you're unfit, walk or swim briskly enough to increase your heart rate and make yourself perspire slightly for 20–30 minutes four to five times weekly.

- Eat fresh fruit and vegetables – and drink their juices – to pep up your immune system, which is among the first bodily systems to suffer when you are stressed and anxious. Celery, carrot and apple juice in equal quantities with 45 ml (3 tbsp) lettuce juice makes an excellent tranquillizer.

- Foods rich in the amino acid tryptophan boost brain levels of the neurotransmitter serotonin, which calms frayed nerves and improves sleep. Good sources include roast beef, lamb, liver, pumpkin seeds, turkey, chicken breast, skimmed milk, Brazil nuts and soya products.

- Herbal relaxant remedies for anxiety include betony, catmint, chamomile, lemon balm, lime flowers, lobelia, rosemary, St John's wort and valerian. You can choose a proprietary product containing an assortment of these, or sip chamomile or lime-flower tea, add sprigs of rosemary to your bath or take capsules of powdered valerian at bedtime.

- Beneficial *Bach Flower Remedies* include Rock Rose for panic, terror and hysteria and Cherry Plum for fear of losing control and of doing dreaded things.

- Useful *aromatherapy* essences include bergamot, chamomile, clary sage, jasmine, lavender, melissa, neroli, patchouli, sandal-wood and ylang ylang.

- Try these homoeopathic remedies for panic attacks. Take every few minutes for up to ten doses:

  o As a first resort: Arnica 30c

  o For paralysing fear: Opium 6c

  o For weakness and trembling after the panic attack has sub-sided: Gelsemium: 6c.

- Practise *Yoga* to control your anxiety and stabilize erratic breathing.

- Try these *acupressure* points:

  o Heavenly Pillar to relieve stress, eyestrain, exhaustion, insomnia and a stiff neck.

  o Sea of Tranquillity for nervousness, chest tension, anxiety and hysteria.

  o Use the Third Eye Point to calm the physical symptoms of anxiety.

- Most importantly, practise full *relaxation* every day and learn to relax in a moment (SEE *pages 266–7*) to cope with unexpected stress and tension.

Drug remedies

○ Antidepressants such as amitriptyline and venlafaxine are more often prescribed nowadays to control anxiety than addictive tranquillizers such as lorazepam and diazepam.

SEE YOUR DOCTOR IF...

- You experience unacceptable levels of anxiety despite home remedies.

■ Carpal Tunnel Syndrome

Carpal tunnel syndrome affects one or both wrists and hands. You may experience pins and needles and numbness in your thumb and next three digits, pains shooting up your forearm and swelling in the part of your hand adjoining your wrist. These symptoms seem worse at night but are relieved by hanging the affected arm over the side of the bed.

The underlying problem is compression of the nerve supplying sensation and movement to the thumb and next three fingers as it enters the hand from the forearm. In doing so, it has to pass through the carpal tunnel, between your wrist bones (or carpus) and a tough layer of overlying connective tissue. Hormonal changes, injury and inflammation can all cause swelling, which presses upon and damages the nerve.

WHAT YOU CAN DO

- Help to prevent carpal tunnel syndrome by seeking prompt medical attention for all wrist injuries and for fluid retention.

- Take medication and exercise as recommended for *arthritis*, if you are a sufferer, to minimize damage to your wrists.

- Take a daily vitamin supplement (SEE *below*).

- Avoid excessive rotational wrist action, for example wringing out heavy washing and any DIY involving the use of screwdrivers.

- Take up a wholefood eating plan with five or more daily portions of fresh fruit and vegetables, including asparagus, carrots, celery, dandelion leaves and parsley, all of which combat fluid retention. Celery and carrot juice go well together: you could juice them in roughly 1:1 proportions and add a handful of parsley or dandelion leaves for extra benefit.

- Carpal tunnel syndrome due to a deficiency of vitamin B6 (pyridoxine) – as a feature of the *premenstrual syndrome* or poor diet – generally responds well to supplements of this nutrient taken in addition to a multivitamin/mineral supplement. Foods rich in B6 include egg white, yeast, spring cabbage and other green leafy vegetables, wheat bran and wheatgerm, cantaloupe melons, lean meat and milk. You are probably better off taking a supplement, however, because pyridoxine is destroyed by heat, contact with light and long-term storage in tins and deep freezers. The recommended daily amount (RDA) is 1.6–2.0 g, although much larger doses are prescribed by nutritionists treating carpal tunnel syndrome and other complaints.

- Other useful nutrients include the whole B complex, vitamin C with bioflavonoids, vitamin E, selenium, zinc, calcium, magnesium, vitamin D and beta-carotene.

- Vegetal (as opposed to mineral) silica derived from horsetail is useful for hormone-linked fluid retention. Other useful diuretics which a medical herbalist might prescribe include broom, heather flowers, juniper, parsley piert and pellitory.

- Apply a cool compress to burning, tingling wrists and add a drop or two of fennel, frankincense, geranium or juniper essential oil.

- Try these homoeopathic remedies four times daily for up to 2 weeks:
  - When there is a great craving for salt: Natrum mur. 6c
  - When the pain is relieved by warmth and rubbing: Magnesium phos. 6c
  - When the pain is severe enough to wake you at night: Aconite 30c

Drug remedies

- Diuretics (water pills) may be prescribed for aggravating fluid retention.
- Simple painkillers and NSAID anti-inflammatories such as ibuprofen may help.
- Hydrocortisone injections into the wrist may bring relief.

SEE YOUR DOCTOR IF...

- Carpal tunnel symptoms persist despite home remedies.
- If you need an operation to relieve the pressure – the sooner you have it, the fewer the risks of serious nerve damage.

■ Depression

Depression can take a number of forms, but the most common feature is a persistent low mood which colours your view of your environment and other people and your ability to cope with them. This differentiates it from 'the blues' due to the *premenstrual syndrome*, for example, and from feelings of sadness, boredom, disappointment, rejection and bereavement grief. Poor self-esteem, guilt and self-blame are invariably present when you are clinically depressed, your sex drive tends to plummet and activities such as socializing, which you normally enjoy, lose their attraction.

Physical symptoms are also common, and include poor-quality sleep, *loss of appetite* or a tendency to comfort eat, lethargy, exhaustion and daytime drowsiness, weight loss or gain and *constipation*. Mentally, you are less alert than usual, have difficulty in concentrating and find your short-term memory and organizing ability badly affected. There is often no apparent cause for depression, although bereavement, a failed relationship or job loss can all trigger it.

WHAT YOU CAN DO

- Reduce stress to a minimum. This may be difficult given your personal circumstances, but depressive illness is invariably caused by one (or several) forms of stress, including childhood and other past traumas. While you cannot alter the past, you can learn, through cognitive behavioural therapy, other forms of psychotherapy and counselling, to deal with it in a way that negates or minimizes its power to harm you.

- Similarly, seek help if needed to resolve relationship problems, money worries, housing difficulties and other causes of ongoing stress.

- Boost your immune system against the debilitating effects of stress – falling prey to infectious illnesses and allergies or, possibly later on, to cancer, while obviously undesirable in themselves, will also impede your efforts generally to relieve depressive symptoms.

- Follow the nutritional advice for *anxiety* (which often plays an important role in depression), including the tryptophan-rich foods, since depression sufferers also need to boost their serotonin levels. However, you should swap the nerve-soothing juice suggested for a high-vitality pep-up drink if you are lethargic and drowsy rather than anxious. Blend equal quantities of unsweetened grapefruit, orange and tomato juice with a handful of watercress and some liquid ginseng supplement (for quantities, SEE label instructions). Serve over ice and decorate with fresh mint.

- Take a multivitamin/mineral supplement with extra B complex (for stress) and zinc, which has been shown in trials to relieve depression in some cases.

- Exercise boosts serotonin levels and releases endorphins in the brain, which revives a low mood and combats depression. Follow the advice for *anxiety*.

- The herbal remedy St John's wort (hypericum) has been shown in clinical studies to relieve mild and moderate depression. Ginseng is often recommended – take in the juice drink above or as a supplement. Herbal teas made from basil, thyme and/or mint may also prove helpful.

- Have a warm relaxing bath or massage using 3–4 drops of bergamot, clary sage, marjoram, neroli, rose, verbena or ylang ylang essential oils. You can also inhale them from an oil burner at home and from a tissue carried with you during the day.

- These *Bach Flower Remedies* are worth trying: Mustard for wretchedness that descends without a known reason, Honeysuckle if you are living with memories rather than in the present, and Gorse or Gentian for loss of hope and feeling that it is pointless to try.

- Depression is always triggered by stress in some form. Relax daily (SEE *Anxiety*).

Drug remedies

o Antidepressant drugs such as the 'tricyclics' group – for example amitriptyline, nortriptyline.

o Selective serotonin re-uptake inhibitors (SSRI) antidepressants such as fluoxetine, sertraline and venlafaxine.

SEE YOUR DOCTOR IF...

- Simple home measures fail to relieve a low mood.

▪ Dizzy Spells

Dizzy spells can be frightening and they cause both accidents and falls. Causes range from *high* or low *blood pressure*, the side-effects of anti-hypertensive drugs and anaemia to low blood sugar, panic attacks and a disturbance of the inner ear.

The last-mentioned is responsible when dizziness takes the form of vertigo – a definitive sensation of movement, as though you or your surroundings are rotating. A viral infection of the inner ear or labyrinth (labyrinthitis), fat-clogged arteries or Ménière's disease are commonly responsible. Links also exist with *migraine* and epilepsy. Accompanying symptoms are likely to include feeling exhausted, nausea and vomiting.

WHAT YOU CAN DO

- Establishing the cause of your dizziness is important, both to rule out more serious conditions and to enable treatment to start. Have regular blood pressure checks, especially if being treated for hypertension, and check with your doctor if you think medication may be responsible for your problem.

- For the sudden onset of a dizzy spell, lie down, loosen all constricting clothing and take the Bach Rescue Remedy.

- Eat plenty of wholefoods to keep your blood sugar within normal limits, including wholegrain snacks, fruit, vegetables, nuts and seeds. Pistachio and cashew nuts and pumpkin seeds are good sources of iron. Oats and oatmeal soothe the nerves and turkey raises your serotonin levels, bringing a sense of calm and lifting your mood.

- Make sure you drink eight glasses of water daily and take isotonic sports drinks if you have been sweating heavily. Water and electrolyte loss affects the highly sensitive labyrinth; dizziness due to a fall in blood pressure is typically seen on sudden rising.

- If you have an ear infection, take antibiotics as prescribed. Dizziness linked to middle ear damage can prove difficult to treat.

- The inner ear, as such, is not usually accessible to herbal remedies, but ginger and the herb betony are often prescribed to relieve dizziness. Useful remedies for the associated nausea and vomiting include ginger as the remedy of choice, while aniseed, black horehound, cassia, chamomile, cinnamon, Irish moss (carrageen) and nutmeg can also work well.

- *Aromatherapy* essences to combat dizziness include chamomile, cinnamon, ginger and nutmeg – and lavender for its deeply comforting, soothing effects upon an irritated nervous system. Anti-nausea essences such as black pepper, chamomile, marjoram and the aniseed-flavoured fennel can all work quickly and effectively too.

- Try these homoeopathic remedies for labyrinthitis. Take once hourly then less frequently for up to twelve doses:

  - When dizziness is made worse by lying down or turning the head sideways: Conium 6c

  - When vomiting is induced by eye movements: Bryonia 30c

  - For dizzy spells in an elderly person due to arteriosclerosis (hardening of the arteries), when they also have *high blood pressure* and *palpitations*, and especially if an aneurysm (bulge in arterial wall) is present, there is also Vanadium 6c. Take twice daily for a month and consult a homoeopath if there is no improvement.

  - For dizziness, especially where there are *fainting attacks*, confusion, mental deterioration, liver problems and the heart feels squeezed within the chest: Vanadium 6c

- *Acupressure* points to relieve dizziness include:

  - Gates of Consciousness

  - Sea of Energy

  - Sea of Vitality

  - Three Mile Point

- Practise *Yoga* and *relaxation* regularly to overcome *anxiety* and panic attacks.

Drug remedies

- Prochlorperazine (Stemetil) is commonly prescribed for dizzy spells.

- Other drugs include hyoscine, beta-histine and the antihistamine cinnarizine.

SEE YOUR DOCTOR IF...

- You suspect *high blood pressure* (or other) treatment may be to blame.
- Your dizziness takes the form of vertigo.
- You are having falls.
- Your dizzy spells persist despite simple treatments.

▪ Headaches and Migraine

Headaches affect us all at some time, and while dental, neck and jaw disorders can be responsible, tension is the most common cause. Tension headaches pulsate, or feel like a 'tight band around the skull'. They are triggered by fatigue, worry and stress, and can be relieved by simple home measures.

Migraines affect around 1 in 10 people and the classical type produces an intense throbbing pain on one side of the head, often above the eye. Classical migraines tend to develop after a 20-minute warning period or aura, with numbness, tingling and/or muscular weakness and visual disturbances such as flashing lights, zigzag lines and halos around lighted objects. Nausea, vomiting, *abdominal pain* and sometimes *diarrhoea* can also feature. Migraine attacks are generally over within 24 hours and are also generally amenable to home treatment.

WHAT YOU CAN DO

- Keep junk snacks and high-fat high-sugar foods to a minimum. Small regular wholefood meals and snacks prevent hypoglycaemia and contain no artificial additives such as nitrates, nitrites and monosodium glutamate (MSG), which have all been implicated in migraine attacks. Other dietary migraine triggers include alcohol, chocolate, cola, pork, onions, garlic, eggs, corn, citrus fruit, tinned figs, wheat, coffee, cheese, pickled herrings (rollmops), chicken livers and broad bean pods.

- For headaches and migraines linked to hangovers, *stomach upsets*, tiredness and tension, try mixing two parts of tomato juice to one of celery. Sip a wineglassful every two hours while symptoms persist.

- Try to keep regular hours and get as much sleep as you need without oversleeping. Sleep deprivation and excess are both linked to migraine attacks.

- From the medical herbalism viewpoint, most migraines are 'cold' (due to excessive blood vessel constriction) and therefore relieved by a *hot compress* to the head. Peripheral vasodilator remedies (SEE *Poor Circulation in the Hands*) such as elderflowers, feverfew, ginger or peppermint are also helpful. Ginger also combats nausea and vomiting, while peppermint eases painful bowel spasm.

- 'Hot' migraines due to excessive vasodilation are relieved by *cold compresses* and a herbal bitter such as celandine, chicory or white horehound, or a relaxant such as chamomile, lime flowers, passionflower, skullcap or valerian.

- Useful *aromatherapy* oils for hot migraine include lavender, lemon balm and rosemary, and for cold migraine gelsemium (yellow jasmine), hyssop and sage. You can inhale the oils and/or add them to the appropriate compresses.

- Tension headaches often respond to old-fashioned smelling salts based on salts of ammonia scented with lavender oil. Interestingly, ammoniac, a gum resin and volatile oil extracted from a plant native to Iran, is a herbal relaxant and peripheral vasodilator.

- Keep tension at bay with regular *Yoga* and *relaxation.*

- Get to work on these *acupressure* points:

  o Bigger Rushing, especially good for hangover headaches.

  o Gates of Consciousness, for headaches and migraines, stiff neck and neck pain.

  o Third Eye Point, good for headaches and eyestrain.

Drug remedies

o Painkillers – paracetamol, aspirin, NSAIDs. Combined paracetamol + metoclopramide (Maxolon), an anti-nauseant, anti-vomiting drug.

o Migraine preventatives, for example pizotifen, beta blockers, for example propranolol, and tricyclic antidepressants, for example amitriptyline.

o Migraine treatments, for example the NSAID tolfenamic acid, are specifically licensed to treat acute migraine attacks. Almotriptan, sumotriptan and others work on serotonin receptors in the brain.

SEE YOUR DOCTOR IF...

- You experience migraines while taking the combined contraceptive pill – it may be responsible.
- Headaches or migraines persist.

■ ME (Myalgic Encephalomyelitis)

Also known as post-viral and chronic fatigue syndrome, ME is thought to affect around 1 in 300 people in the UK. It is three times commoner in women and usually develops between the ages of 20 and 45 – or, in children, between 13 and 15 years, although it can develop earlier.

The most common feature of ME is severe physical and emotional exhaustion, unlike anything experienced previously, largely unrelieved by rest and unexplained by physical or emotional exertion. Many, although not all, attacks develop after a viral illness such as glandular fever or *flu*, and a recurrent *sore throat* and swollen glands are common features of the condition. Others you may experience include muscular and joint pain, *headache*, pallor, cold hands and feet, pins and needles and numbness in the limbs, inability to sleep or persistent drowsiness and symptoms similar to *irritable bowel syndrome*. You may also feel disorientated, find your memory and concentration affected and have difficulty with everyday tasks such as decision making, understanding the spoken and written word and simply collecting your thoughts. You may also suffer from *depression, anxiety*, panic attacks, mood swings and an increased susceptibility to stress of all kinds.

There are no specific tests for ME, which is, therefore, diagnosed by default, but a positive attitude and home remedies can relieve the symptoms and promote recovery.

WHAT YOU CAN DO

- The approach generally recommended to ME sufferers combines three measures:

  - Graded exercises, for example walking and swimming, with gradually progressive increases in aerobic exercise. This applies only to those with mild to moderate symptoms which permit some physical exertion; the idea is that inertia (although inevitable, at least initially) eventually aggravates ME and that small regular amounts of exercise help to condition the body. Routines need to be tailored to individual needs and are best drawn up in co-operation with a physical therapist and/or physician.

○ Pacing – this approach to exertion alternates activity with rest to encourage increased stamina and avoid the boom or bust scenario in which maximum effort is followed by near-collapse.

○ Cognitive behavioural therapy (CBT) – a branch of psychotherapy increasingly practised in the UK and based on the belief that thinking habits can fuel health problems. CBT seeks to improve symptoms, coping strategies and day-to-day functioning.

• Wholefoods rich in immune-boosting antioxidants and free of artificial chemicals are of huge importance in ME. Two theories of its cause include *intestinal thrush* and an abnormal immune reaction following a viral infection. Pomegranate juice may help ME sufferers with recurrent *sore throats* – gargle with it, then drink it.

• *Acupressure* points to treat ME target its chief symptoms and boost your immune defences:

○ Sea of Vitality relieves a whole host of ME symptoms, particularly extreme fatigue, muscular weakness, dizziness, confusion and irritability.

○ Shoulder Well relieves fatigue, *anxiety*, mood swings, *headaches*, nervous problems and cold feet and hands.

• A homoeopathic remedy specifically for ME, to be taken every 12 hours for up to 3 days, is China 30c.

Drug remedies

○ Immunoglobulin injections have been given to boost the immune system.

○ Sometimes antidepressant drugs are helpful.

○ Other approaches specifically target joint and muscle pain, irritable bowel symptoms, etc.

SEE YOUR DOCTOR IF...

• You think you may have ME. Other causes for profound tiredness, etc. need to be ruled out.

▪ Memory Problems

Failing memory can be caused by nervous tension, fatigue, psychological or emotional trauma and age-related dementia, which is caused by plaque deposits and/or poor circulation to the brain. Centres controlling cognitive function and emotional control suffer accordingly.

Whatever the cause, short-term memory suffers first. You may repeat remarks and questions many times over and forget what you had for breakfast, for example. Long-term memory remains intact for far longer and it can be frustrating to retain a clear picture of childhood events and not the times and places of imminent appointments.

WHAT YOU CAN DO

• To prevent or minimize mental decline, keep your brain active with crosswords, word puzzles and quizzes.

- Remain involved with life and other people – play cards or Bingo, meet friends, dance, read books and newspapers and watch/listen to plays and the news.

- A wholefood diet, stress reduction and therapies to relieve the effects of stress can all help. The need for a healthy blood supply to the brain, which is always paramount, becomes even more pressing when clogged cerebral arteries may be responsible for cognitive loss. This means avoiding saturated dietary fat as far as possible and using cold-pressed vegetable oils containing cis-linoleic acid and other polyunsaturates instead.

- The best source of protein is oily fish – you could aim at a 100 g (3½ oz) portion three or four times weekly. The essential fatty acid EPA (SEE *Salmon* in *Nutritional Medicine*) and the related DHA are both vital brain nutrients, so take a fish oil supplement if you are a non-fish eater.

- Lean poultry and eggs are also good sources of protein, essential for the replacement of worn-out or damaged tissues in the brain and elsewhere.

- Dietary supplements could be beneficial: a multivitamin/mineral complex, plus fish oil if required (SEE *above*), vitamin B complex to combat stress, vitamin E for improved arterial health and vitamin C with bioflavonoids for their potent antioxidant properties. A little extra selenium and zinc could be added to boost immunity and lift a low mood (SEE *Depression*).

- Regular gentle 'effort' exercise commensurate with general health increases the serotonin and endorphin levels and peps up the blood circulation to the brain. If your poor memory is due to *depression* or stress, you would benefit similarly *and* find an outlet for accumulated tension.

- Herbal ginkgo biloba extracts have been shown to improve memory, alertness and general mental function through their beneficial effects upon the brain's blood circulation and energy metabolism. They may also act as antioxidants, further slowing down the brain's decline with age.

- Add a few drops of essential oil of rosemary to an oil burner or bathwater – it is a physical relaxant and may enhance the brain's cognitive function.

- Useful *Bach Flower Remedies* include Clematis for someone who is absent-minded and dreamy and has problems in concentrating. Walnut assists in the adjustment required for transition or change, for example when a partner dies or goes into hospital, children leave home or a house move looms.

Drug remedies

- Donepezil, galantamine and rivastigmine do not delay, halt or cure Alzheimer's dementia, but they may improve some of the early symptoms.

- Memantine (with a different mode of action) is prescribed for moderate to severe Alzheimer's dementia.

- In Europe, ginkgo biloba extracts are extensively prescribed for age-related dementia.

SEE YOUR DOCTOR IF...

- Even the mildest symptoms persist despite home remedies.

▪ Sciatica

If you have sciatica, you will be familiar with the nagging 'toothache-like' pain in your buttock and/or down your leg, which is aggravated by sneezing and coughing. Standing may be more comfortable than sitting, but walking may be very painful. You may also have *lower backache* or a history of low back injury and experience pins and needles, numbness and muscular weakness or wasting.

Like *carpal tunnel syndrome*, sciatica is a form of neuralgia or nerve pain caused by compression – in this case of the body's largest nerve, the sciatic. This leaves the lower end of the spinal cord, passes under the buttock muscles and then goes down the leg to the foot, supplying the entire lower limb with sensation and movement.

This nerve can be damaged or pressed upon by a prolapsed disc or bony outgrowths from the last two lumbar and/or first three sacral vertebrae, creating symptoms in the muscles and skin areas of the buttock, thigh, lower leg and foot supplied by the affected fibres.

WHAT YOU CAN DO

- Try to prevent sciatica from developing or worsening by seeking medical treatment for all lower back injuries.

- Follow medical advice – rest flat, for instance, for the prescribed time, then ease back *gently* into action.

- Lose excess weight and keep it off!

- Accept physiotherapy if offered; practise the exercises between sessions.

- Take regular gentle exercise such as walking, swimming and aquarobics (but check first with your doctor or therapist).

- Learn how to lift heavy or awkward objects safely (keep your back straight and bend your knees).

- Eat wholefoods to counteract any tendency to gain surplus pounds. They will also keep your bowels regular – straining can be excruciating when you have sciatica.

- Oat cereal for breakfast supplies energy throughout the morning and acts as a nerve tonic.

- Herbal remedies would include relaxants, for example chamomile, lavender, lemon balm, lobelia and rosemary, analgesics such as aconite, gelsemium, Jamaica dogwood and wild lettuce, and nerve restoratives such as Korean ginseng, lavender, oat preparations, squaw vine, St John's wort and vervain. You could perhaps sip chamomile tea flavoured with sprigs of lavender or lemon balm and take a commercial aconite preparation and a daily ginseng supplement.

- There are a wealth of homoeopathic remedies for sciatica. Here are three of them: take hourly for up to ten doses, or half-hourly if the pain is acute:

  ○ For pain shooting down the right leg to foot, with some weakness and numbness, the pain being aggravated by damp cold weather: Colocynth 6c

  ○ For lightning-like pains in the right leg worsened by coughing and improved by heat: Magnesia phos. 6c

  ○ For pain in the left leg aggravated by cold and heat, with increasing stiffness and difficulty in walking: Carbon sulph. 6c

- Beneficial *acupressure* points include:

  ○ Commanding Middle

  ○ Sea of Energy

  ○ Sea of Vitality

- Gentle *Yoga* asanas that help to strengthen back muscles when the acute pain has passed include the Grip, Knee to Chest, Kneeling Pose, Shoulder Stand and Twist.

Drug remedies

○ Painkillers – from aspirin, paracetamol and paracetamol + codeine to opiate-linked dextropropoxyphene, dihydrocodeine and tramadol.

○ NSAID anti-inflammatories, for example ibuprofen, celecoxib.

○ Muscle relaxants, for example diazepam, methocarbamol and carisopradol.

○ Steroid injections.

SEE YOUR DOCTOR IF...

- The pain persists despite exercises and home remedies.
- You develop muscle wasting or other signs of protracted nerve entrapment.

▪ Shingles

If you have had an attack of shingles, you will remember the rash and pain you experienced somewhere on your chest or lower body or, if you were particularly unlucky, on your face, scalp or genital area. You may have felt feverish and unwell for a few days and felt pain in the body area supplied by the affected nerve before noticing a rash. Small red spots would then have appeared, soon developing into itchy *blisters*. Most people recognize a shingles rash, but not everyone realizes that the pain (postherpetic neuralgia) can continue long after the spots have gone.

Shingles is caused by an infection of the root of a sensory nerve by the chickenpox virus, Herpes zoster. The virus, which has often lain dormant for decades, spreads along the nerve from its origin in the spinal cord or brain, causing symptoms.

Shingles is not infectious, nor is it dangerous unless it affects the ophthalmic nerve supplying the front of the eye (for which specialist treatment may be required). There is no truth to the old wives' tale that a rash breaking out on both sides of the spine can be fatal if it meets around the front. However, shingles is an unpleasant illness and you need to rest and recover.

WHAT YOU CAN DO

- Shingles is especially likely to develop following a debilitating illness such as cancer, a bereavement, a fall or some other trauma. Bearing this in mind, although you cannot actually prevent shingles, you *can* consciously fortify your immune system against it (and other) infections.

- Eat lots of fresh fruit and vegetables, raw or freshly juiced wherever possible. You could have oat porridge for breakfast with fresh fruit; a large daily salad, fruit, vegetable crudités, seed and nut snacks and stir-fried vegetables including carrots, pumpkin, squash, tomatoes and broccoli with your protein-based meal.

- A restorative drink recommended for shingles sufferers consists of 250 ml (½ pint) each of carrot and celery juice, mixed with 10 ml (1 dsp) parsley juice and some liquid Korean ginseng (SEE package label for quantity).

- Herbal remedies for shingles include damiana, ginseng, oat preparations and St John's wort as nervous restoratives and for the rash a linseed poultice or a cold compress soaked in an infusion of calendula, chamomile, horehound, horsetail or lavender or a tincture of St John's wort.

- Essential oils of chamomile, geranium, lavender and lemon can be added to a carrier oil as for a massage and smoothed gently into the spots or into the soles of the feet.

- Try these *acupressure* points:

    ○ Gates of Consciousness for pain and inflammation in the upper half of the body.

    ○ Sea of Energy to boost your immunity.

    ○ Sea of Vitality

- Combat nervous exhaustion with the relevant *Bach Flower Remedies.*

- And use *Yoga* and regular *relaxation* to regain vigour and relieve stress.

Drug remedies

○ The anti-viral drug aciclovir tablets.

○ Aspirin, paracetamol with and without codeine, NSAIDs such as ibuprofen.

○ Gabapentin, which specifically targets neuropathic (disordered-nerve) pain, is often prescribed for postherpetic neuralgia (pain following shingles).

○ Calamine lotion.

SEE YOUR DOCTOR IF...

- You need prescription medicines.
- The rash and pain are not relieved by home measures.

▪ Tinnitus

Traditionally known as 'ringing in the ears', tinnitus causes more distress than many other ailments. How you cope with it depends to an extent upon your usual ability to handle stress and your willingness to use diversionary aids (SEE *below*). Some sufferers claim to be driven nearly insane by the constant buzzing, hissing and whining noises, so the sooner the cause is established and you start to take remedies, the better.

Almost any disorder of the mechanical parts of the ear, or its nerve, can be responsible. Common causes include wax in the ear passage, irritation of the auditory nerve by aspirin and blockage of the Eustachian tube, a narrow passage running between the middle ear (which conducts sound waves from the eardrum inwards) and the back of the nose above the soft palate. Catarrh or thick mucus formed during a *common cold, sinusitis* or throat infection can form a small plug in the Eustachian tube, altering the pressure in the middle ear chamber and causing muffled hearing, sound echoes and tinnitus.

WHAT YOU CAN DO

- Take home remedies for *colds, flu* and other conditions causing nasal congestion.

- A mucus bubble can sometimes be dislodged by the Valsalva manoeuvre: breathe in, close your mouth, pinch your nostrils and attempt to blow through your nose. Stop if you experience pain – your eardrum may be inflamed, in which case antibiotics should be considered.

- Cut back on aspirin: if you are on regular 75 mg doses to keep your blood thin, see your doctor about the tinnitus.

- Keep the lining membranes of your throat and airways healthy with plenty of fresh fruit and vegetables. Eat broccoli, rich in vitamin C, calcium and magnesium, and pumpkin, rich in alpha- and beta-carotene, daily for a week or two and/or drink several glasses daily of freshly squeezed orange juice, rich in vitamin C and bioflavonoids. Flavour with a little freshly grated ginger root for added benefits to the inner ear (SEE *Dizzy Spells*).

- Medical herbalists treat accumulated ear wax with daily drops of warmed olive oil to soften the plug, check the eardrum for damage, then syringe the ear, if appropriate, with a solution of the astringent Septfoil, marigold or witch hazel. They may treat middle ear problems with olive oil eardrops containing extracts of garlic or mullein flowers.

- Inhale decongestant essential oils such as cedarwood, eucalyptus, pine and tea tree. Nerve calmers for incessant tinnitus include chamomile, clary sage, lavender, rose, rosemary and ylang ylang.

- Acupressure:

  o Bigger Stream relieves earache and ringing in the ears.

  o Use Wind Screen for painful ear conditions generally.

Drug remedies

o Antibiotics and decongestants as appropriate for *colds, flu, sore throat* and *sinusitis.*

o There are no specific drug treatments for tinnitus, although an antihistamine such as cyclizine is sometimes prescribed if a disorder of the inner ear's labyrinth or vestibule is suspected.

SEE YOUR DOCTOR IF...

- You wish your ears to be checked for wax.
- Home remedies are ineffectual. The cause may need to be investigated and you may need a hearing test.
- You would like to try one of the sound distraction devices which are available to compete with and block out the unwanted noises.

14

Ailments of Muscles, Joints and Bones

---

* Arthritis * Bruising and torn muscles * Fibrositis
* Lower backache * Osteoporosis * Problem feet
* Sprains and strains * Upper back pain

■ Arthritis

Arthritis can start unexpectedly or develop in a previously injured joint. You'll recognize the symptoms if a sufferer – stiff, painful, possibly swollen joints and restricted movement.

Most of us develop a degree of osteoarthritis (OA) as we age, mainly in the weight-bearing joints of the hips, knees, ankles and lower spine. Triggers include lack of exercise, overuse of the affected joints (for example frequent, prolonged jogging on hard surfaces) and poor nutrition.

Rheumatoid arthritis (RA), commoner in women, is an immune system defect and generally affects the smaller joints of the fingers, wrists and elbows. Gout, commoner in men, is due to a build-up of uric acid crystals in joints such as the big toes and knees. Causes include defective metabolism of uric acid (a protein by-product excreted in the urine), kidney disorders and certain diuretic drugs. Flare-ups cause crimson swollen joints which may be agonizingly painful.

WHAT YOU CAN DO

- Minimize your risks of developing arthritis by shedding surplus weight.

- Fortify your immune system (which is overtaxed by chronic inflammation, whatever the source) by dealing effectively with stress and cutting out saturated fat and all accessible 'E numbers' (i.e. steer clear of processed foods and junk snacks).

- Try cutting out salt, sugar, white flour products and cow's milk (substitute goat's milk products).

- Obtain protein from oily fish such as salmon, kippers, tuna and sardines; vegetarian combinations of pulses, legumes, grains, seeds and nuts; fat-free poultry; and lean red meat (avoid the last if it aggravates your symptoms).

- Eat *at least* five 100 g (4 oz) portions of antioxidant-rich fruit and vegetables daily. Aim at one 'raw foods only' day a week – muesli with fresh or dried fruit, seeds and nuts, live organic goat yoghurt, salads, tofu, bean dishes and reduced fat cheese are all good choices. Add some wafer-thin slices of raw salmon or tuna, Japanese-style, if liked.

- If a gout sufferer, try eliminating strawberries, citrus fruit, alcohol, red meat and tomatoes.

- Two recommended juice recipes to relieve acute arthritis symptoms: 500–1,000 ml (1–1¼ pt) of freshly squeezed celery juice daily. For gout, add a few crushed celery seeds, which increase the elimination of uric acid from the body. Or 125 ml (5 fl oz) each of carrot, beetroot and cucumber twice daily.

- Take a multivitamin/mineral combination, plus extra B vitamins and supplementary evening primrose oil and fish oil. Green-lipped mussel extract also reduces inflammatory arthritis symptoms. Glucosamine and chondroitin sulphate supplements are also very helpful.

- Useful herbal remedies include cider vinegar, honey, pollen and garlic; devil's claw (which also boosts uric acid elimination); and chamomile or melissa tea to reduce stress and relax muscular spasm.

- Add *aromatherapy* essences of cypress, juniper and/or pine to a warm bath, or make into a hot compress or a massage oil.

- Try gentle *Yoga* asanas to retain joint flexibility and aid stress reduction.

- Practise *relaxation* and meditation regularly to calm body and mind.

Drug remedies

- Paracetamol, either alone or combined with codeine.

- Aspirin (though not for gout); non-steroidal anti-inflammatory drugs (NSAIDs) such as ibuprofen.

- For gout, high doses of an NSAID such as indomethacin for acute attacks and specific anti-gout drugs such as sulfinpyrazone or allopurinol to control uric acid formation between attacks.

- Oral and injected steroids for OA and RA.

SEE YOUR DOCTOR IF...

- You develop stiff, swollen, painful joints for a fortnight or longer.
- Simple remedies are ineffectual.

▪ Bruising and Torn Muscles

You develop a bruise after a blow or fall damages soft tissue, releasing blood into the surrounding area. A red mark appears immediately after impact; over the following hours or days, it turns dark blue, greenish blue then yellow before finally fading as the blood is broken down and removed by immune defence cells. Throughout this time the bruised area feels tender to the touch and sometimes a small (harmless) lump remains behind after the tissues have healed.

A muscle tear is equally if not more painful. The injured muscle swells, hurts and may develop extensive bruising. You will find your use of it restricted until the muscle fibres have been repaired. Vigorous sports are the commonest cause of torn muscles, followed by excessive exercise and accidents.

WHAT YOU CAN DO

- Cut the risks of bruising and torn muscles by wearing appropriate protective clothing for sports (for example elbow, knee, facial and crotch guards, helmets and gloves).

- Increase your muscular stamina gradually – avoid sudden, violent or excessive exercise.

- Take advice from a sports or fitness instructor on the advisability of warm-up exercises.

- Keep your muscles in healthy trim with regular stretching and safe aerobic routines.

- Eat wholefoods, protein and fresh fruit and vegetables to repair minor soft tissue damage and encourage healthy repair. Bioflavonoids, found in citrus fruit and other natural sources, together with vitamin C, maintain strong capillary blood vessels throughout the body. This reduces the risks of local blood loss and bruising if a soft tissue injury occurs.

- Drink this bioflavonoid-rich juice twice daily: place all the flesh and juice you can extract from one fresh grapefruit and one fresh orange in a blender, scraping the inner pith well and including fragments of the white membrane. Blend with some crushed ice, a handful of fresh mint and a little unprocessed honey if you wish.

- Low-fat proteins supply amino acids to replace worn-out cells without increasing your cholesterol count. Choose oily fish, lean poultry and soya foods with phyto-oestrogens and other nutrients which maintain small blood vessel health.

- Herbal remedies for bruising include arnica and comfrey creams and ointments. Do not use on broken skin because they speed healing so effectively that debris or dirt can become trapped in the wound.

- Freeze some distilled witch hazel in an ice cube mould and apply to the bruised area or torn muscle, or wrap in a cloth so that the melting ice cube trickles directly onto the injury.

- A handful of crushed daisies applied directly to a muscle tear or bruise, or made into a compress or poultice (SEE *page 26*), can bring great relief.

- Wintergreen ointment relieves torn muscles.

- Smooth massage oil containing cypress, lavender or mint *aromatherapy* oil into bruises. Use fennel, rosemary or thyme for sore torn muscles.

- Homoeopathic remedies:

  o Immediately after tearing a muscle, then hourly for up to six doses and four times daily for up to three days: Arnica 30c

  o If pain persists, take Rhus tox. 6c four times daily for up to seven days.

Drug remedies

o Simple analgesia – paracetamol, codeine, aspirin – and NSAIDs such as ibuprofen.

SEE YOUR DOCTOR IF...

- Pain, swelling and/or bruising are severe – bone injuries must be ruled out.
- You develop a haematoma – a swelling containing released blood immediately below the skin.
- Home remedies bring no relief.

▪ Fibrositis

If you suffer from fibrositis, you will know exactly what it feels like, although doctors have argued for years about the nature of this condition and even questioned its existence. However, most experts now agree that it refers to the inflammation of small muscular nodules which develop between the shoulder blades when the upper back muscles become stressed and tense. Small buds of muscular fibres 'pop' through weak spots in the surrounding membranous envelope, where they become pinched and short of blood. A tissue reaction sets in, causing inflammation, and the nodules cause a toothache-like pain in the surrounding tissues and in the adjacent shoulder and arm, too, if they press on a nerve.

Signs of fibrositis include a detectable muscular knot between the upper spine and shoulder blade; pressure upon it greatly aggravates the discomfort. The pain tends to be worse on hot windy days and after exercise. Vigorous exercise of the upper back and shoulder muscles can quell the pain for a little, but it inevitably returns.

WHAT YOU CAN DO

- Avoid straining your shoulder muscles by carrying or trying to move awkward heavy weights.

- Keep your shoulder muscles healthy with gentle daily stretch exercises of the upper limbs and torso. Swimming in a heated pool reduces tension build-up in the affected muscles.

- Check the positions in which you spend long hours regularly. Hunching over a computer or other machinery may be aggravating your discomfort – check your chair height, etc. for maximum health and safety.

- Cover up after exercising and avoid perspiration cooling on your uncovered upper back.

- Eat wholefoods as recommended for *bruising and torn muscles* or for *arthritis.*

- Raw foods and juices offer relief for rheumatic pain: a useful juice combination combines 350 ml (12½ fl oz) carrot juice with 110 ml (4 fl oz) spinach juice. Drink twice daily, immediately after juicing.

- Old country remedies for *arthritis* include sleeping in a thin-walled sack of fresh fern; a hot poultice of fresh-picked ferns or cabbage; and a compress utilizing 1 litre (1¾ pts) water in which you have soaked a finely chopped onion, plus one handful each of fresh broom, chamomile, heather and/or lavender, left to steep until cool or at body temperature.

- Useful *aromatherapy* oils include chamomile, lavender, marjoram and origano. Use to make a massage oil or add to bathwater or an oil burner.

- Homoeopathic remedies to take 3 hourly for up to 2 days:

  ○ Rhus tox. has been shown to be as effective as NSAIDs in relieving fibrositis.

  ○ For pain and stiffness when pain gets the person up at night and makes them bad-tempered: Chamomilla 6c

  ○ For pain in the neck and down the arm aggravated by movement and cold dry easterly winds but soothed by pressure: Bryonia 30c

- *Acupressure* points to relieve shoulder tension include:

  ○ Gates of Consciousness

  ○ Heavenly Rejuvenation

  ○ Outer Arm Bone

  ○ Shoulder Well

- Combat physical and mental tension with regular *Yoga* and *autohypnosis*. Beneficial *Yoga* asanas include the Corpse, Knee to Chest, Plough and Shoulder Roll. If you have a back disorder, osteoporosis or other health complaint, check first with your doctor about your fitness to do these exercises.

Drug remedies

○ Paracetamol, and paracetamol + codeine combinations relieve fibrositis pain temporarily, but NSAIDs such as ibuprofen (by mouth and as a locally applied cream or spray) are more likely to help.

Carisopradol may be prescribed for severe muscular spasm.

SEE YOUR DOCTOR IF. . .

- You suffer from persistent or recurrent pain in the upper back and shoulders which is unrelieved by home measures.

▪ Lower Backache

Lumbago (lower back pain) can interfere with every aspect of your life and it generally results from over-vigorous exercise or incorrect lifting. Hauling on a heavy weight at ground level, by bending from the waist and heaving, strains the lumbar spine and aggravates the nearby spinal nerves.

A strained or torn muscle hurts immediately then goes into further painful spasm. The fibrous ligaments that bind the vertebrae can also become damaged, producing severe pain in the spinal joints and muscles.

A (more serious) slipped disc results when the fibrous cushion between to adjacent vertebrae slips out of position and presses on a nearby nerve, causing severe lower back pain while lifting or shortly afterwards. Sitting or walking a few steps may be impossible until the inflammation subsides.

Spondylitis (sharp spicules of bone growing out of the edges of the lumbar vertebrae pressing on nearby nerve fibres) causes chronic backache, as does osteoarthritis of the lumbar or sacral spine (SEE *Arthritis*).

WHAT YOU CAN DO

- Learn to lift correctly: keep your back straight, bend your knees and lift slowly. Do not try to shift heavy furniture or similar objects unaided.

- Rest is a priority for lower back pain. Either lie on the floor, for maximum support to the lower spine, or in bed, with a chopping board or similar placed under the mattress below your lower back.

- A hot shower or bath can do much to relieve lower back pain, and swimming in a heated pool as soon as you are able will prevent further stiffening of the spine and muscular weakness developing from underuse.

- Try this core muscle exercise. On all fours, allow your stomach to sag downwards. *Gently* pull in your stomach, moving your navel closer to your spine. Avoid deliberately using six-pack or other muscles. Hold this position for 4 seconds and repeat 20 times. As your technique improves, hold for 20 seconds and practise while sitting or standing.

- Useful herbal preparations include devil's claw and willow, containing salicylates, the natural form of aspirin. Herbal thyme or chamomile tea help, due to their muscle relaxant actions. Make a poultice with 15 mls (1 tbsp) of linseed oil mixed with 5 drops of pine or thyme *aromatherapy* oil, heat gently and leave in place for 20 minutes; repeat daily as required. Make a massage oil using 10 mls (1 dsp) carrier oil and 5–6 drops of angelica, juniper, pine or thyme essential oil; use for a gentle massage of your lower back twice daily.

- For despondency for lower backache which you feel will never be resolved, try the *Bach Flower Remedies* Gorse or Larch.

- Useful *acupressure* points include:

  o Womb and Vitals to relive lower backache, *sciatica* and muscular tension

  o Sea of Vitality, which also relieves the tiredness which frequently accompanies chronic back pain

- Regular *relaxation* and *autohypnosis* are useful for combating the *depression* that many chronic backache sufferers experience.

Drug remedies

o Paracetamol alone or combined with codeine, and NSAIDs such as ibuprofen.

SEE YOUR DOCTOR IF. . .

- You experience persistent pain anywhere in your back. You may need physiotherapy or some other form of manipulation, or an exercise regimen to prevent the pain and stiffness from becoming chronic.

▪ Osteoporosis

If you are a middle-aged or more mature woman, you may have been diagnosed with osteoporosis (brittle bone disease) or suspect that you have it after suffering one or more fractures. The most important cause of serious fractures in older people, osteoporosis is due to a loss of minerals from the skeleton, making the bones progressively brittle and liable to break. Every adult starts to lose skeletal calcium (and associated elements) from around the age of 30, but only around 3–5 per cent of women and 1 per cent of men go on to develop brittle bone disease. You are several times more at risk if you are female because the fall in the hormone oestrogen levels that occurs at the menopause hastens calcium loss.

A major symptom of osteoporosis is experiencing a bony fracture after a comparatively minor injury – fractured neck of the femur (a hip fracture) after a fall is typical. Others include a loss of height due to crush fractures of the spinal vertebrae and, developing slowly over many years, a 'dowager's hump' (humped back).

WHAT YOU CAN DO

- Reduce the risk of developing osteoporosis by maintaining bone strength throughout your life. This involves regular weight-bearing exercise such as walking, gentle jogging or dancing – ballroom dancing, in fact, is suitable for all ages and keeps many older people of both sexes sprightly, fit and fracture-free into (and beyond) their eighties. Regular stretching – an anatomically correct 'pull' of muscles upon the bones anchoring them – especially to the spine and lower limbs also helps to strengthen the bones' substance.

- Have a bone-density scan to see whether you are at risk, especially if close older female relatives have suffered (SEE ALSO *page 298*).

- Eat wholefoods and eliminate tea, coffee and cola drinks; reduce alcohol intake to 2 units a day maximum. Phyto-ostrogens found in soya products, sprouted seeds and grains are beneficial. Fresh fruit and vegetables (and other antioxidant food sources) fortify the immune system against ageing. Maintain a regular intake of low-fat calcium-rich foods such as skimmed milk and its products and green leafy vegetables. Other useful nutrients include magnesium, copper and phosphorus.

- Take a multivitamin/mineral supplement, with additional calcium, magnesium, silica and copper if your diet is lacking these nutrients.

- Herbal and *aromatherapy* remedies are essentially the same as those recommended for the *menopause*. Fractures are encouraged to heal more quickly with daily applications of comfrey cream or ointment. (Comfrey is also called knitbone.) Apply to unbroken skin only.

- If you sustain a fracture, take the Bach Rescue Remedy straight away to reduce the shock and stress.

- *Yoga* is extremely helpful in combating stiffness, pain and immobility (all of which contribute to falls in later years). Useful asanas include the Corpse and Salutation to the Sun. If you have a back disorder, osteoporosis or other health complaint, check first with your doctor about your fitness to do these exercises.

Drug remedies

○ Hormone replacement therapy (HRT).

○ Drugs affecting bone metabolism, for example etidronate and alendronate, which increase new bone formation and bone mass (density).

○ Calcium, vitamin D and magnesium supplements.

SEE YOUR DOCTOR IF...

- You wish to discuss HRT.
- A high street pharmacy bone scan indicates osteoporosis.
- Your mother and other close female relatives have suffered from this condition.

■ Problem Feet

Painful feet can make your life a misery. Causes range from the easily controllable – ill-fitting or unsuitable shoes, excessive standing or walking – to the easily remediable – *warts* and *verrucas, corns* and *calluses* – to those requiring treatment, for example bunions, gout (SEE *Arthritis*), flattened arches (flat feet) and reduced blood supply (SEE *Poor Circulation in the Feet*).

Another common cause you may not have considered, or your doctor may not have diagnosed, is plantar fasciitis, which often responds to home measures. The underlying disease process is inflammation of the plantar fascia – the tough fibrous sheet of connective tissue deep under the skin in the sole of the foot. The acute form affects people of all ages and produces pain under the heel when you are standing or walking. The pain can extend along the inner edge of the sole, and acute plantar fasciitis is sometimes linked to more generalized inflammatory conditions such as gout. More common in people aged 40–60 years, the chronic form occurs in the same area as the acute, but is less severe. Also known as 'policeman's heel', it has no known link with other inflammatory disorders.

WHAT YOU CAN DO

- Rest is a major requirement for plantar fasciitis, although this is sometimes difficult when it means time off work. Nevertheless, acute inflammation is unlikely to subside until anti-inflammatory treatment has started to work.

- Footbaths may help by delivering remedies directly to the sore area and cool compresses soothe an inflamed sole. Weight reduction is also important, if applicable.

- Eat wholefoods, including plenty of fresh fruit and vegetables with their high antioxidant content, to strengthen your immune system and help to overcome inflammation. This is especially important if your plantar fasciitis is linked to a more generalized inflammatory condition such as gout or rheumatoid *arthritis*. Aim to include as many raw foods as possible and drink juices daily. You could try freshly squeezed grapefruit juice, including a little pith and membrane for their bioflavonoid content, blended with liquorice juice (made by dissolving a solid liquorice stick in water) for its anti-inflammatory action.

- Useful anti-inflammatory herbs include those with a significant salicylate (natural aspirin) content such as birch, black haw, meadowsweet, willow bark and wintergreen. You can take some of these by mouth or make them into cool foot baths or compresses. Liquorice has a steroidal effect, as do ginseng (both varieties) and wild yam.

- Make a massage oil using pimiento oil, warm it slightly and apply it gently to the painful area. Cover with a *hot compress* and keep it in place for 20 minutes morning and night to relieve acute symptoms.

- Useful homoeopathic remedies, to be taken 4 hourly for up to 3 doses, include:

  ○ For feet that ache after excessive standing or walking: Arnica 30c

  ○ For burning soles, aggravated by walking: Graphites

  ○ For soles that are painful to step on, when there is tightness and pain in one or both Achilles tendons: Muriatic ac. 30c

- Try these *acupressure* points:

  ○ Bigger Stream when your feet are swollen.

  ○ Calf's Nose for swollen, rheumatic or arthritic feet.

Drug remedies

○ Simple analgesia such as paracetamol, paracetamol + codeine.

○ NSAIDs such as ibuprofen applied locally as a cream or spray, and taken by mouth.

○ Hydrocortisone injections into the sole to reach the inflamed plantar fascia.

SEE YOUR DOCTOR IF...

• Home remedies bring no relief.
• You think you may have a more generalized inflammatory condition.

▪ Sprains and Strains

If you have ever sprained your ankle, you will know that it can be as painful as a cracked bone or fracture. It happens when a powerful force is exerted on a joint at a particular angle. In the case of the ankle, the lateral ligament supporting the outside of the joint can be partly torn away from the bones into which it is inserted, in a simple sprain, or entirely detached from them if the sprain is severe. The tendons and ligaments of the back, trunk and limbs, on the other hand, are more prone to strain, a lesser injury often resulting from uncustomary exercise or effort.

A simple sprain causes a joint to swell painfully, and slight bruising may appear. The swelling and pain are more marked with a severe sprain; the *bruising* is often intense and widespread around the damaged tissues, and an X-ray often shows that a fragment of bone has been ripped from the anchor site. A strain makes the affected tendon or ligament and its adjoining muscle sore to the touch; all these injuries greatly hamper movement, and rest is usually required for healing to occur.

WHAT YOU CAN DO

- Reduce the risks of sprain or strain injury by shedding surplus weight; wearing support boots where recommended, for example for hill or fell walking, especially if you have weak ankles; and avoiding sudden bursts of vigorous, uncustomary exercise, for example line dancing.

- If you suffer an injury, follow any simple exercise or rest regimen prescribed.

- Protein-rich foods are needed to supply the amino acids required for replacing and rebuilding damaged tissues. Eggs, pulses, nuts and seeds, fish, lean meat and poultry and vegetarian recipes balancing legumes, cereals, grains, seeds and nuts are all useful. Sources of tryptophan-rich protein sources (SEE *Depression*) also increase serotonin levels, which help to reduce pain and relax muscles in spasm (for example after an injury).

- Juices: try those recommended for *arthritis* and take a multivitamin/mineral supplement, evening primrose oil, fish oil and glucosamine to strengthen and heal injured tissues.

- Herbal remedies: arnica cream applied to the injured area, or arnica solution, used for making a cold compress. Comfrey, also known as knitbone, applied as a cream, ointment or tincture also reduces swelling, bruising and pain, and promotes healing. Thyme tea is an anti-spasmodic and encourages blood flow to an injured area, promoting tissue repair.

- Useful *aromatherapy* oils include cajeput, niaouli and rosemary. Add them to bathwater and have a long soak. Chamomile essential oil reduces painful muscular spasm in the injured area.

- *Bach Flower Remedies*: use Rescue Remedy straight after an accident to reduce pain and shock. Alternatively, Star of Bethlehem, a component of Rescue Remedy, can be used alone.

- Homoeopathic remedies:

  - Try Natrum carb. 30c every 12 hours for up to a week.

  - For strained or pulled muscles, immediately after injury: Arnica 30c every hour for up to 6 doses, then 4 times daily for up to 3 days.

  - For pain that persists despite Arnica, use Rhus tox. 6c 4 times daily for up to 7 days.

Drug remedies

- Simple analgesia – paracetamol with or without codeine, aspirin, NSAIDs such as ibuprofen.

- In the case of a severe sprain, stronger painkilling drugs may be required.

SEE YOUR DOCTOR IF...

- You suspect a severe sprain – an X-ray may be needed to distinguish this injury from a fracture.
- Simple home remedies do not bring relief or cure.

▪ Upper Back Pain

If you have experienced upper backache, you may agree with other sufferers on the pain's toothache-like quality. It's a burning, gnawing sensation usually located between the shoulder blades or higher up near the base of the neck. Arthritic changes and spondylitis in the upper trunk vertebrae are frequently to blame. The joint spaces tend to narrow as we age and small spikes of bone (spicules), developing around the edges of the joints, become inflamed, causing pain and limited movement.

WHAT YOU CAN DO

- In addition to wholefoods, fresh raw fruit and vegetables and their juices, include oily fish and green-lipped mussels in your diet as sources of protein. (The latter can be found in many supermarkets with a wet fish counter.) Try to limit animal protein portions to 100g (4 oz) three to four times weekly and seek other sources in tofu, reduced fat cheese and vegetarian combinations of grains, pulses and nuts.

- Also cut down stringently on refined carbohydrate (high-GI) foods (SEE *page 6*) and junk snacks with a high refined-sugar content. All these items are likely to contribute extra acid waste after digestion and are best avoided by *arthritis* sufferers.

- The antioxidants present in plant foods have an anti-inflammatory effect, so eat regular portions of broccoli, pumpkin, blueberries, spinach, citrus fruit and tomatoes (include the latter two only if your symptoms are not aggravated by them).

- Regular stretching and bending exercises can help by easing muscle spasm and reducing the pressure of spicules on adjacent nerves. Hot showers, baths, compresses and swimming in a heated pool can also help to reduce painful inflammation.

- Cod liver oil, green-lipped mussel extract, omega-3 fatty acids and evening primrose oil ease arthritic inflammation of many types.

- Traditional herbal remedies include honey and cider vinegar, garlic and pollen, chamomile and capsaicin. Alfalfa raw, or as tablet supplements, is also recommended. The traditional approach aims to improve the circulation in and around the joint, thereby encouraging the removal of irritant toxic waste with locally applied rubifacients (superficial circulation boosters) such as cayenne, the mustards, horseradish, ginger and prickly ash.

- *Aromatherapy* essence of aspic (old English lavender) or ordinary lavender can be used. Add 4–5 drops to a warm bath and soak thoroughly. After drying, with the area still warm, add 5 drops of either oil to 10 mls (2 tsp) sweet almond or soya oil, and massage it gently (or have it massaged) down the side of the tender upper spine.

- Specific homoeopathic remedies for spondylitis, to be taken 4 times a day for up to 14 days, include:

  - For tenderness at the back of the neck and over the backward pointing spines of the upper back vertebrae, for when the chest feels tight and the patient is weak and shaky: Agaricus 6c

  - For shooting pains up the spine and into the head and neck, when the neck feels on fire: Picric acid 6c

  - For a tender upper spine, with *headache* behind the forehead, with a frontal *headache* when the person's limbs feel numb and they have wind: Argenum 6c

  - For a tender upper spine, with *headache* behind the forehead: Argentum nitrum

Drug remedies

○ Simple analgesia (for example aspirin, paracetamol, either alone or combined with codeine).

○ NSAIDs, for example ibuprofen.

SEE YOUR DOCTOR IF...

• The symptoms fail to clear up within a few days.
• Home remedies do not help.

15

Miscellaneous Ailments

- Blood sugar imbalance • Croup • Earache
- Insomnia • Itchy red eyes • Measles
- Motion sickness • Teething

▪ Blood Sugar Imbalance

You may have experienced hypoglycaemia (low blood sugar) after taking in large quantities of sweets, biscuits, sweetened drinks or other sugary foods. The symptoms of shakiness, sweating, nausea, faintness and a racing pulse are caused by the huge slug of insulin released into the bloodstream in response to your snack, which drives the temporarily raised blood sugar down to unusually low levels.

High-GI foods (high-glycaemic index foods with a high sugar but low or absent fibre content) can have the same effect. Familiar examples include white wholegrain bread and white pasta, short grain white rice, toasted rice cereals, instant potato, lettuce, red cabbage, peppers, marrow, watermelon and dried dates. If you frequently overindulge in sugary snack binges, the pancreas gland which produces insulin can become overtaxed, responding less efficiently to your usual diet. This, in turn, can increase your risk of suffering from diabetes in the future.

High blood sugar (hyperglycaemia) is unlikely to bother you unless you have been diagnosed with diabetes. Type I diabetes usually starts in your teens or twenties and is insulin-dependent, i.e. you need to inject insulin regularly to keep your blood sugar within acceptable limits. Type II (maturity onset) diabetes starts in middle age and is normally controlled by diet alone or diet plus medication.

WHAT YOU CAN DO

- Reduce your intake of sugary foods and snacks and eat more low-GI foods whose high fibre content reduces the rate at which sugar is released into the bloodstream. Examples include multi-grain bread (white and brown), heavy fruit breads, brown and wild rice, other wholegrains, tabbouleh, pearl barley, whole-wheat pasta, oats/porridge, unsweetened muesli, high-fibre wheatbran cereal, sweet potato, okra, peas and beans, broccoli, aubergines, apples, oranges, pears, bananas, honey, jam, soya milk and its products.

- If you suffer from diabetes, maintain your blood sugar within advised limits by eating according to the above lists and consistently reducing your intake of refined high-GI carbohydrates.

- If you suffer from hypoglycaemia, try to eat low-GI foods at every meal and to include some if you do decide to snack on high-GI foods.

- Chromium is a component of the body's glucose tolerance factor and can be beneficially added as a supplement to a wholefood low-GI diet for the control of hypoglycaemia. It also helps reduce insulin dependence and both total and LDL cholesterol levels in diabetics. It can be found in mulitivitamin/mineral supplements or taken in addition to one.

- Try to follow every aspect of any plan mapped out for you by your GP or diabetic clinic adviser. This includes diet, daily exercise, drug remedies and attendance at your regular diabetic clinic.

- Herbal bitters regulate the release of insulin and glucagon (another carbohydrate-linked hormone) by the pancreas and in this way can aid the control of both hypoglycaemia and diabetes (this dual action is possible because of bitters' adaptogenic properties (SEE *Ginseng, pages 21–2*).

- These homoeopathic remedies, to be taken four times daily for up to 14 days, may aid the control of diabetes:

  - For symptoms worsened by nervous exhaustion, for example grief, nervous tension: Phosphorus ac. 6c

  - For symptoms that include digestive upsets, weight loss, bedwetting and weakness: Uranium nit. 6c

  - Where there is skin irritation, *depression* and restlessness: Codeinum 6c

  - Where there is also gout: Nattrum sulph. 6c

  - Where symptoms include perspiring, cold bad-smelling feet and overall weakness: Silicea 6c

Drug remedies

- Insulin.

- Sulphonylurea drugs such as glibenclamide, glicazide and glipizide.

○ Biguanide drugs such as metformin.

○ Thiazolidinedione drugs such as pioglitazone and rosiglitazone.

○ Prandial glucose regulators such as nateglinide and repaglinide.

○ Alpha-glucosidase inhibitors such as acarbose.

SEE YOUR DOCTOR IF...

- You experience frequent hypoglycaemic attacks despite home measures.
- You suspect that you may be suffering from diabetes at any age.

▪ Croup

Most mothers know the child's condition croup. It is due to inflammation and swelling of the larynx or voice box and follows (or occurs together with) a feverish *cold* or *sore throat*. The child has a whistling high-pitched *cough* and stridor – crowing, grunting and wheezing due to the larynx's narrowed interior. Epiglottitis, similar to croup, also produces stridor and a high fever, and is caused by bacterial infection of the epiglottis – the lid of tissue over the opening of the larynx which prevents fluids and solids from going down the wrong way.

Both croup and epiglottitis are potentially serious and many hospitals admit babies and small children overnight when brought into A and E with stridor. A few hours in a steam tent, with assisted breathing, generally relieves an acute attack. You can apply steam in the home to treat a croupy *cough*; but you must remain on the lookout for signs of the condition worsening (SEE *pages 312–13*).

WHAT YOU CAN DO

- During a coughing attack, take the child into the bathroom or kitchen, close the windows, leave the extractor fan off and turn on all the hot taps.

- Keep the child's room humidified with bowls of water (out of reach of children and animals).

- Reduce the fever by removing the clothing apart from the pants. Sponge the face and body with tepid water.

- Give cooling drinks – water, fruit or vegetable juices if liked – or an ice lolly to suck. Make your own healthy variety with a freezer lolly kit, using a favourite fruit, for example blueberries or strawberries, puréed and diluted with a little water/juice and sweetened if necessary with honey. Frozen banana has novelty appeal and ensures a source of carbohydrate, fibre, potassium and other nutrients and a little fluid. Peel and cut a banana into chunks, dip it in a little fruit juice or runny honey, coat it with carob powder (natural chocolate substitute), foil-wrap and freeze on lolly sticks.

- While convalescing from croup (or before, if acceptable), offer a little homemade soup, for example pumpkin, broccoli and potato or carrot. Blend to remove lumps and enrich with cow's, goat's or soya milk and grated cheese if liked.

- Keep the child's immune defences generally boosted by encouraging them to eat a wide range of fresh foods and to drink some plain water every day (in addition to fresh juices, milk, tea, etc.).

- Demulcent herbal remedies (which soothe inflamed mucous membranes) can prove helpful. For older children, look for marshmallow and comfrey lozenges or teas (*check age-relevant details on package*) or give the child a liquorice stick to suck (obtainable from health stores). (NB Overuse of liquorice can cause *diarrhoea.*)

- Benzoin is the traditional essential oil for the treatment of laryngitis and croup; others include lavender, sandalwood and thyme. Add a few drops to a steam inhalation or make up a massage oil and rub it gently into the child's chest.

- Try these homoeopathic remedies specific for croup:

  - For a child who wakes in the night, coughing and distressed at breathing difficulty: Aconite 30c at once, and repeat once after 30 minutes if the child is not asleep.

  - If this does not bring relief, give Spongia 6c and Hepar sulph. 6c alternately every hour for up to three doses each.

Drug remedies

- Paracetamol or nurofen to help reduce temperature.

- Antibiotics if bacterial infection is present.

> **SEE YOUR DOCTOR IF...**
> - The child's breathing or other symptoms worsen.
> - Simple remedies bring no relief.

▪ Earache

You can suffer from earache at any age, although the younger you are, the more common the problem. You may run the risk of barometric trauma if you fly a lot or go deep-sea diving, but the most usual cause is infection of the middle ear, the cavity in the skull enclosed by the eardrum to the outside, and the small membranous window leading to the inner ear which houses the balance organs. Babies and children are especially likely to experience this condition, known as otitis media and characterized by a painful and inflamed eardrum.

Otitis media can start for no apparent reason or follow upon an upper airways infection such as a *cold, tonsillitis* or other form of *sore throat*. The symptoms to watch out for are sharp throbbing pain deep within the ear (infants usually cry and scream unremittingly), together with a fever, *headache* or *sore throat*. The affected ear may also discharge pus. Should this build up, due to lack of treatment, it may press upon the eardrum until it bursts.

WHAT YOU CAN DO

- Try to prevent ear infection by drying your ears thoroughly after bathing or swimming.

- Cover your ears with a woolly hat or ear muffs in severely cold or windy weather.

- Use home remedies or seek medical attention for a child's persistent catarrh or *sore throats*, which can predispose it to otitis media.

- Breastfeed your baby during the first few months of life. Studies have shown that antibodies obtained from mother's milk dramatically cut the risks of childhood middle ear infection.

- Boost your (or your child's) immune defences with a wholefood eating plan containing fresh fruit and vegetables daily. Most children will drink orange juice: buy the real juice rather than the 'juice drink' and/or get them to scrape out the flesh or an orange or grapefruit (sweetened with honey if necessary) to ensure an intake of bioflavonoids and vitamin C. Other beneficial juices include grape, carrot, blueberry and cranberry; mix in a little lettuce juice to calm an earache sufferer fractious with pain.

- Useful herbal preparations include alfalfa (also good, raw, in salads), astragalus, cat's claw, echinacea and ginseng (both varieties). You can also make a tepid infusion of calendula or chamomile (from a tea bag or handful of fresh herb) and use to soak a small wad of cotton wool before inserting gently in the ear.

- *Aromatherapy* essence of calendula, chamomile, clove or marjoram can be used to make a little massage oil. Warm gently and smooth around the ear and behind over the mastoid prominence (the part of the skull behind the ear, identifiable as a smooth knobble behind the earlobe). Rub the chest with eucalyptus, geranium, pine or tea tree oil (in a massage oil) or use other home remedies for catarrh and nasal congestion (SEE *Colds and Sore Throats*).

- Useful *acupressure* points include:
  - Bigger Stream – also good for *tinnitus*
  - Ear Gate
  - Listening Place
  - Reunion of Hearing
  - Wind Screen

Drug remedies

- Antibiotics are essential for middle ear infection, usual choices being amoxicillin alone, or amoxicillin + clavulanic acid (potentized form).

- Paracetamol, aspirin and non-steroidal anti-inflammatory drugs (NSAIDs) such as ibuprofen.

○ Antibiotic/corticosteroid eardrops, for example those containing neomycin, polymyxin B, hydrocortisone.

SEE YOUR DOCTOR IF...

• Earache is severe or persistent, as a perforated eardrum can seriously affect hearing and the infection can spread into the air spaces of the mastoid bone. Mastoidiitis is a serious condition often requiring surgery and can even lead to meningitis.

▪ Insomnia

We have all had one or a series of sleepless nights, but true insomnia is difficulty in getting to, and/or remaining, asleep over an extended period of weeks and months. You are probably left frazzled, irritable and jet-lagged, with poor concentration and short-term memory, and daytime drowsiness. Most chronic insomniacs will agree that there is nothing more annoying than fighting the urge to sleep during daylight hours, only to spend all night fretting, tossing and turning.

Physical causes include coming off tranquillizers or sleeping medication, poorly controlled pain, late pregnancy discomfort, bladder or prostate problems demanding frequent bathroom visits, a blocked nose, menopausal flushes and night sweats, *sleep apnoea, restless legs* and a heart or lung problem causing breathlessness or a *cough*. A heavy meal late at night can also be responsible, as can coffee, tea and other caffeine drinks, alcohol (especially if taken in excess), an uncomfortable bed, a snoring, muttering partner or an overheated, stuffy room.

More often, emotional problems are responsible. These range

from grief, *depression* and *anxiety* to reading or watching disturbing books or TV programmes just before bed. One of the most common causes is the fear of being unable to sleep or of recurrent bad dreams.

WHAT YOU CAN DO

- Take a positive view that your insomnia can be resolved.

- Rectify any causes under your control such as a lumpy mattress, an airless bedroom and late night caffeine, cheese, heavy meals and/or alcohol.

- Ask a restless or snoring partner to seek help for their ailment. Meanwhile, catch up on some sleep with a few nights in a spare bedroom.

- Swap alcohol for a milky drink at bedtime. Disregarded by many as too simplistic to work, a hot milky drink provides calcium and the amino acid tryptophan to calm the nerves (SEE *Depression*) and induce peaceful rest. Ovaltine or Horlicks can be added to hot milk or a teaspoon of honey can be added to increase the availability of the tryptophan.

- Sip herbal teas such as chamomile, lime flower, melissa or vervain last thing at night. If unsuccessful, try preparations of cowslip, passionflowers, skullcap, St John's wort or valerian. A medical herbalist might prescribe Jamaican dogwood, lady's slipper or wild lettuce.

- Essential oils for insomnia relief to add to your bath or a massage oil include benzoin (especially when external worries are responsible), bergamot (which also relieves *depression*) and clary sage, a profound relaxant never to be combined with alcohol as it can cause nightmares.

- Learn and practise *relaxation* and/or *autohypnosis* daily. Combine with one of the other home remedies to potentiate the effect of each.

- Learn and practise *Yoga* regularly to stretch and soothe tense under-exercised muscles and calm a troubled mind. Asanas specifically recommended for insomnia include the Cobra, Corpse, Locust, Mountain and Posterior Stretch.

Drug remedies

○ Benzodiazepine sedatives, for example nitrazepam.

○ Non-benzodiazepine sedatives, for example zolpidem, zopiclone.

○ Other over-the-counter products such as Nytol.

SEE YOUR DOCTOR IF...

- You suffer from nightmares or similar sleep disturbances, grief, *anxiety* or *depression*.
- Self-help tips and home remedies for physical causes (for example *restless legs, sleep apnoea*) do not bring relief. Your doctor could prescribe medication for bladder weakness (for example), refer you to a sleep laboratory for *sleep apnoea*, or review your current pain relief, heart or lung medication.

▪ Itchy Red Eyes

Itchy red eyes provide two sources of discomfort. You look (and therefore feel) far from your best, and the persistent irritation and soreness interferes with work and leisure. The most common causes are airborne pollutants, pollen or some other allergen and infection. If the former, the sclera (whites) of the eyes become bloodshot and the eyes water and itch; in the case of infection, bacteria are nearly always to blame and pus appears too. Secreted from the eyes together with tissue fluid, the cream-coloured, yellow or green pus can interfere with vision, especially when thick and purulent, and glue the eyelids together while you are asleep. This can be frightening, especially for children, but careful bathing of the lids soon restores normal vision.

WHAT YOU CAN DO

- Protect your eyes with sunglasses in hot windy weather if prone to *hayfever*.

- Wear goggles or an industrial mask if dealing with noxious substances.

- Keep your flannel, sponge and eye makeup scrupulously clean – never borrow or lend these items.

- Avoid contamination spreading if one family member has bacterial conjunctivitis. It is extremely infectious and personal items such as face towels and flannels need to be kept separate.

- Boost your immune system against allergy and infection with wholefoods, regular exercise and *relaxation*. Blueberries are known traditionally – and have been proven clinically – to strengthen blood capillaries throughout the eye, and encourage ophthalmic health. Include a large handful in your five (or more) 100g (4 oz) daily portions of fresh fruit and vegetables. You can eat them in pies and tarts (sweetened with dried fruit such as apricots or a little honey); in smoothies, yoghurt and fresh juice drinks; and in muffins, muesli and porridge (the oats would be especially beneficial, because they have a mildly tranquillizing effect on nerves irritated, in this instance, by eye discomfort).

- Vitamin A is also vital to eye health. You can obtain this from any of the beta-carotene rich foods mentioned in Part I, or take it as a supplement, together with a basic multivitamin/mineral supplement. (Large quantities of vitamin A can be toxic; this does not apply to its pro-vitamin form.)

- Herbal remedies for irritated and/or infected eyes include blueberry extract taken by mouth and infusions of chamomile, cornflower and marigold for making cool compresses which are applied to the forehead and closed eyelids. Eyebaths of the plant eyebright (*Euphrasia officinalis*) are a common treatment for bacterial eye inflammation. You can also make cool eye compresses by adding a drop or two of chamomile, fennel or parsley essential oil to cold water.

- If you have nothing else to hand, place cool slices of freshly cut cucumber on your eyelids and rest for half an hour. Cool wrung-out tea bags or a cold poultice of finely chopped parsley rubbed and squeezed to release some juice also work very well.

- Useful *acupressure* points include

  o Drilling Bamboo

  o Facial Beauty

  o Four Whites

  o Heavenly Pillar

Drug remedies

o Corticosteroid eye drops (for allergic conditions), for example prednisolone.

○ Antibiotic eyedrops and ointment, for example chloramphenicol, gentamicin, polymyxin B.

SEE YOUR DOCTOR IF...

- Home remedies bring no relief after 4–5 days. Untreated eye irritation, especially the infective variety, can damage the eyes and permanently impair vision.
- Urgently if your eyes have been irritated with a noxious substance or fumes.

▪ Measles

If your baby or child catches measles, you will probably find that it has been passed on by other children or family members with whom they have been in contact. It is a highly infectious viral illness spread by *coughs* and sneezes, and one bout normally confers immunity for life, although subsequent attacks occasionally occur. Until the age of 6 months, babies are protected by their mothers' antibodies; but they do need to be immunized if they are to avoid the disease later on.

The incubation period of 10–11 days is followed by the pre-rash phase and the child is infectious from the first day of this phase until 5 days after the rash appears. During the 3–4 day pre-rash period, the child starts off with a *sore throat*, high temperature, *cough*, red running eyes and/or a runny nose, followed within 24 hours by the appearance of Koplik's spots (raised white salt-like spots inside the mouth), which confirm the measles diagnosis.

The rash phase lasts 2–3 days. The spots are dark red, flat or slightly raised and appear first on the forehead, around the hairline and behind the ears, then spread downwards to rest of the body. The temperature returns to normal as the rash fades, and the spots turn brownish and scaly before disappearing.

WHAT YOU CAN DO

- Have your child immunized.

- Boost the child's immune defence system with fresh fruit and vegetables which are rich in antioxidants. If salad and lightly cooked vegetables are unacceptable, offer fruit and freshly squeezed juices.

- Homemade orange juice, grapefruit juice or lemonade sweetened with honey supply vitamin C and bioflavonoids. Or try tomato juice, or naturally sweet carrot and/or beetroot juice, adding some lettuce for its nerve-calming properties. (You might benefit from a glass yourself, if your child has been fractious and kept you awake all night.)

- Reduce fever with elderflower or lime-flower tea, or a preparation of willow bark. (SEE ALSO *herbal remedies for Colds, Coughs and Sore Throats/Tonsillitis.*)

- Diffuse eucalyptus or tea tree oil throughout the sickroom, using a burner or spray. From four years onwards, reduce fever by sponging with two drops of bergamot and/or chamomile added to ½ litre (1 pint) of tepid water.

- Homoeopathic remedies include the Morbillinum nosode (made from measles-infected tissue or fluid) to reduce risks of catching the illness:

  - Pre-rash phase – give 2-hourly for up to 10 doses – for *cold* symptoms and high temperature: Aconite 30c or Belladonna 30c

○ For a child who is feverish, won't drink, is tearful, has thick green catarrh, a *stomach upset* and a night *cough* and the light hurts their eyes: Pulsatilla 6c

○ Rash phase – give 4-hourly for up to 10 doses – rash slow to appear, child irritable with high fever and thirst, hacking cough which aggravates a *headache*: Bryonia 30c

○ For a rash slow to clear – spots turn purple: Sulphur 6c

Drug remedies

○ Paracetamol to soothe *headaches* and general discomfort and reduce fever. Aspirin may be given to children over 16 years.

○ An antibiotic if the child's throat shows signs of bacterial infection.

SEE YOUR DOCTOR IF...

• Fever persists or the child still feels ill after the rash fades.
• *Earache* develops, or the eye inflammation, *sore throat* or *cough* are especially troublesome.

▪ Motion Sickness

Motion sickness may be a trivial complaint, but if you are a sufferer, you will know how it can ruin the part of a holiday or trip spent travelling. The chief symptoms, nausea and vomiting, usually disappear shortly after the motion ceases, but a really bad attack can leave you feeling ill for up to 24 hours afterwards, especially if your vomiting has been profuse and you have become dehydrated.

Undoubtedly the worst situation for poor travellers involves the kind of travel over which you have no control. Buses usually stop along the way and cars can draw up at a few seconds' notice, but relentless coach drivers and train, ship and air journeys all cause intense misery.

Motion sickness is due to a disturbance of the balance mechanism in the inner ear (SEE *Dizzy Spells*), and tends to be aggravated by visual irritation, for example gazing at the swiftly approaching road, expecting to feel sick, petrol and other smells, a hot and stuffy atmosphere and a terror of vomiting in public.

WHAT YOU CAN DO

- Parents sometimes take fizzy drinks on journeys to make their children vomit (thereby getting the problem out of the way!) This causes unnecessary suffering because drug remedies and home treatments can prevent nausea from developing in the first place and transform an anticipated nightmare into an enjoyable experience. Drug remedies especially should be taken exactly as prescribed, for example with avomine (SEE *page 325*) take 1 × 25 mg tablet (for an adult) at bedtime before long journeys or 1–2 hours before short journeys.

- Other preventive measures include eating a small dry meal before travelling and sipping mineral water or isotonic (mineral-balanced) sports drinks during the journey to avoid dehydration.

- Keep petrol and other odours to a minimum and windows open where possible; air cabin crew can adjust overhead lighting and air conditioning to suit individual passengers.

- Either close your eyes or avoid watching passing traffic, telegraph poles, etc. *Never* try to read on a jolting journey.

- Keep old-fashioned eau de Cologne or smelling salts available to ward off nausea.

- A wholefood diet rich in antioxidants helps to maintain the inner ear and digestive organs in balance. Foods to avoid for 24–48 hours prior to travel include alcohol, strong tea and coffee, processed foods and junk snacks and all types of fat. Use a cold-pressed vegetable oil or polyunsaturated margarine if essential for spreading or cooking.

- Ginger, aniseed and fennel all combat nausea. Sip the teas or, in an emergency, try ginger biscuits or ginger ale, aniseed balls (or seeds) or a piece of raw fennel. Powdered ginger capsules work well, and lime-flower and lemon balm teas calm anxiety linked to travel. Hot or chilled mint tea settles the stomach after vomiting and removes the unpleasant taste.

- Add a few drops of the *aromatherapy* essences of any of the above or of lemon, marjoram or thyme to your bath or a cool forehead compress, or keep the vials handy to sniff whenever required.

- *Acupressure* works well for motion sickness. The points to work on include:

    ○ Inner Gate

    ○ Intermediary

    ○ Severe Mouth

    ○ Three Mile Point

Drug remedies

○ Anticholinergic drugs such as hyoscine, available as tablets and transdermal patches.

○ Antihistamines such as promethazine, available as tablets.

SEE YOUR DOCTOR IF...

- Over-the-counter medicines and home treatments do not work.
- Nausea and sickness persist for more than 12 hours after motion ceases.

▪ Teething

Teething is blamed for a variety of babies' ailments, including fever, *stomach upsets* and incessant crying. It is, in fact, quite painful, and while there is no reason *why* it should trigger *diarrhoea*, a high temperature or *cold* symptoms, it so often occurs together with these minor disorders that some sort of causal relationship appears certain.

Most babies start teething at around the age of 6 months and have usually cut all their milk teeth (8 incisors, 4 canines and 8 molars) by the end of their third year. The small flaps of skin which are pushed aside by the arrival of the molars (larger teeth at the back) are normal, and they come away from the gum. Sore red gums, dribbling more than usual, crying, irritability, a mild fever and gastrointestinal symptoms – regurgitating recently swallowed food, refusal to eat or drink and mild *diarrhoea* – are all common.

WHAT YOU CAN DO

- You can prevent much of the misery of teething by accepting that a degree of discomfort is inevitable. Extra fluids and tepid sponging help to keep the temperature down, while extra-soft food minimizes gum soreness. Tolerance of a baby's increased irritability and disturbed sleeping pattern will help both your child and you! Lots of cuddles and soothing remedies also bring relief.

- Useful foods (depending on the child's age) include antioxidant sources to reduce the painful inflammatory reaction. Sieved or puréed carrots and/or their juice, pumpkin and broccoli (or the soups made from the boiled vegetables blended with some of their cooking water and milk), soya milks and yoghurts (if suitable to a particular child) all help.

- For protein, minced turkey and other sources of the amino acid tryptophan help to repair damaged gum tissue and increase blood levels of the mood mediator serotonin (SEE *Depression*), which lifts a low mood, improves sleep and blunts the perception of pain. Breast milk also supplies tryptophan, and the supply is increased if you take a high-carbohydrate snack (sandwich, honey plus yogurt, etc.) half an hour before the feeding session.

- Bathe the baby's face and dab their inflamed gums with chilled water (this can also be used to introduce remedies to the mouth and jaws).

- Rest and *relaxation*, a remedy to aid sleep if very fractious, and gentle massage of the scalp, neck and shoulders can soothe screaming attacks.

- Herbal remedies include catnip or chamomile tea which can be suitably flavoured and drunk, or added a few teaspoons at a time to other foods or dab them, when chilled, onto the sore gums. Medical herbalists sometimes prescribe a weak infusion of linden, which you can add to your child's bottle. Alternatively (or also), give the child a piece of chilled carrot, apple or marshmallow root to gnaw on (stay around to check that it does not cause choking).

- Make a cold compress with a small square of gauze folded and dipped into chilled water containing a drop or two of essential oil of catnip, chamomile or clove. Apply to the sore gum area.

Drug remedies

○ Bonjela or similar gum preparations.

○ Other medicines directed at constitutional upsets such as electrolyte solutions for bowel looseness and to combat or prevent dehydration, and/or paracetamol or ibuprofen to reduce pain and fever.

SEE YOUR DOCTOR IF...

- Vomiting, *diarrhoea* and/or other symptoms persist despite home remedies.

First Aid

■ Anaphylactic Shock

CALL AN AMBULANCE

There is no specific first aid measure for anaphylactic shock, an acute allergic reaction to *insect stings*, certain foods such as peanuts, sesame seeds, shellfish and eggs, and to certain drugs. It affects the entire body, dilating the blood vessels, which leads to a profound drop in blood pressure, and narrowing the airways.

The symptoms, which can start within seconds, include swelling of the face, mouth and tongue (which further hampers air intake), widespread red skin blotches and difficulty in breathing which can range from a tight chest to severe wheezing and gasping for air, accompanied by distress and panic. *Unconsciousness, shock and death will follow unless the condition is promptly treated.*

WHAT YOU CAN DO

- The casualty needs a life-saving injection of adrenaline, so the first priority is to call an ambulance, saying you suspect anaphylactic shock and stating the trigger if known.

- Check whether the casualty is carrying the necessary medication – people allergic to bee or wasp stings, for example, may carry a syringe or auto-injection of adrenaline for self-administration. If so, help the casualty to use it. If they are unable to do so and you have been trained to use an auto-injector, give it yourself.

- If the casualty is conscious, get them into a sitting position. This will make it easier for them to breathe. Loosen any tight clothing, especially around the neck. Ask them to take slow deep breaths – it can help to do so yourself and get them to breathe with you.

- Reassure and calm them and treat them for *shock*.

- Monitor the casualty's consciousness level, breathing rate and pulse regularly and be ready to start cardiopulmonary resuscitation (*CPR*) should this be necessary.

- If the casualty loses consciousness, open their airway and check their breathing. Be prepared to give rescue breaths and chest compressions (see *CPR*) if required. If the casualty is breathing, place them in *the recovery position*.

▪ Blisters

Blisters are bubbles of fluid (blood serum) which form below the outer skin layer due to local tissue damage. The most common cause is friction to the hands or feet from uncustomary manual tasks or ill-fitting shoes. Heat, for example *burns and scalds*, and irritating chemicals can also be responsible.

WHAT YOU CAN DO

- Remove or avoid the underlying cause.

- Bathe the blister(s) with herbal or homoeopathic calendula or hypericum solution, pat dry with clean gauze and either expose to the fresh air or cover with an adhesive dressing (keep the adhesive pad away from the blister's surface to avoid tearing).

- Don't prick a blister or remove the overlying skin protecting it from infection.

- Don't pick at loose skin if the blister bursts – bathe and dress as above and change the dressing daily until the blister has healed.

- If practicable, take the dressing off at night in order to help the blister dry out.

SEE YOUR DOCTOR IF...

- Your blisters are slow to heal or recur.
- Your blisters become inflamed and/or ooze blood or pus.
- Your blisters were not caused by pressure or chafing.
- You have diabetes.
- Other symptoms develop.

▪ Burns and Scalds

Most minor burns and scalds happen in the home, but they can also take place outside around a barbecue or campfire and in the workplace. Touching the edge of a hot plate or splashing boiling water over your hands causes acute pain and a bright red skin mark. Deeper burns usually cause *blisters* and hurt for longer than superficial ones. Full thickness burns, which damage the underlying flesh, look charred and grey, but may be relatively painless if nerve endings have also been destroyed. The fluid loss associated with them can lead to *shock*.

WHAT YOU CAN DO

- Take the heat out of the burn straightaway – run cold water over it for at least 10 minutes. Use cold milk or other safe liquids if no water is available (but not ice).

- If clothing or other material is stuck to the burned skin, leave it in place. Seek medical attention.

- Once the burn has cooled, gently remove clothing or any other objects that may constrict the area if the injury swells.

- Do not apply creams or lotions, but cover the burn with a sterile non-adhesive dressing or any clean non-fluffy material and bandage loosely in place.

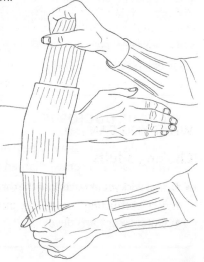

- Place a drop or two of Bach's Rescue Remedy on the casualty's tongue.

- If the burn is severe, take the casualty to hospital. Watch for symptoms of shock and be ready to start *CPR* if the casualty loses consciousness.

- For minor burns and scalds, take paracetamol or a non-steroidal anti-inflammatory drug (NSAID) such as ibuprofen to ease the pain. Aloe vera gel or lavender essence applied to the burned area speeds the repair process, relieves pain and soothes the itch that can develop as the skin heals. Never pop *blisters*.

▪ Choking

CALL AN AMBULANCE.

Choking is caused by obstruction of the windpipe by a fragment of food or a foreign body. The airway is interrupted and *unconsciousness* or death can result if the obstruction is not removed. Babies and young children are particularly prone to choking, either on food such as a sweet or peanut or on some object they have put into their mouths. Symptoms include coughing, going red and having difficulty in speaking.

WHAT YOU CAN DO

Choking adults

- Do not stick your fingers into the casualty's mouth. If you can see the object obstructing the airway, pick it out with your finger and thumb.

- If the casualty is coughing, encourage them to continue. If their *cough* is weak or they cease to breathe, give back slaps. Bend them forwards, stand behind them and slap their back firmly five times between the shoulder blades with the flat of your hand. Then check their mouth to see whether you have dislodged the obstructing object.

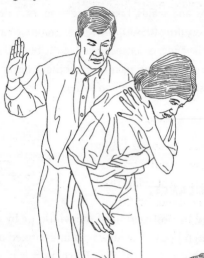

- If this fails, make them bend forwards and, still standing behind them, put your arms around them. Clench your fist, with your thumb inwards, and place it just below their ribs between the navel and breast-bone. Holding your fist firmly with your other hand, pull inwards and upwards five times. This is known as an abdominal thrust.

- If this does not dislodge the object, continue with five back slaps followed by five abdominal thrusts. If the blockage has not cleared after three of these sequences, call an ambulance. If the casualty loses consciousness, be prepared to perform *CPR*.

For a choking child aged 1–7 years

- If the child is coughing, encourage them to continue.

- If this does not work, stand or kneel behind the child (depending on their height), bend them forwards and deliver five back slaps between their shoulder blades. Check their mouth to see whether the object has been dislodged.

- If this is unsuccessful, use chest thrusts. Clench your fist, with your thumb inwards, and place it just below the breastbone. Holding your fist firmly with your other hand, pull in sharply up to five times.

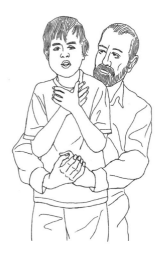

- If this fails, try abdominal thrusts. Place your fist against the child's upper abdomen, just above their navel, hold it firmly with your other hand and pull sharply inwards and upwards up to five times.

- If this does not work, continue with five back slaps, five chest thrusts and five abdominal thrusts. If the child is still choking after three of these sequences, call an ambulance. If the child loses consciousness, be prepared to perform *CPR*.

For a choking baby under 1 year

- The baby may be coughing, crying or unable to make any noise whatsoever. Immediately place them face down along your forearm, with their head below the level of their chest and supporting their body and head. Give their back five slaps with the palm of your hand.

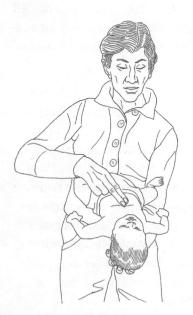

- If this does not work, try chest thrusts. Place the baby face upwards on your forearm, securely supporting their head. Place two fingertips on the lower half of their breastbone, just below nipple level, and thrust downwards five times.

- If this does not dislodge the object, repeat the sequence of back slaps and chest thrusts (never try abdominal thrusts on a baby under 1 year). If after three sequences the baby is still choking, call an ambulance. If they lose consciousness, be prepared to perform *CPR*.

■ CPR

CALL AN AMBULANCE.

Rescue Breathing

Rescue breathing is the first part of a life-saving technique called cardiopulmonary resuscitation – CPR. It is used on an unconscious casualty who has stopped breathing. Blowing your own expired air into their lungs provides them with a vital supply of oxygen. The second stage of CPR is chest compressions (SEE *page 340*). (If a casualty has choked, use chest compressions straightaway.)

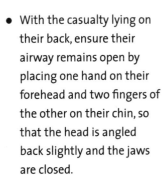

- With the casualty lying on their back, ensure their airway remains open by placing one hand on their forehead and two fingers of the other on their chin, so that the head is angled back slightly and the jaws are closed.

- Pinch their nostrils closed with thumb and index finger and open their mouth. Take a deep breath and place your lips on their lips. Try to form an airtight seal. Blow steadily into their mouth until their chest rises. This should happen in around 2 seconds.

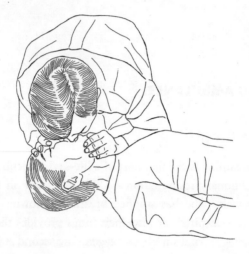

- Keeping their head tilted back, turn your head to see whether their chest falls. If their chest has risen and fallen, then effectively a breath has been taken. If this does not happen, try again to a total of five times.

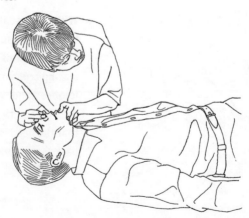

- Once you have achieved two effective breaths, stop the rescue breathing and check the casualty for signs of circulation – coughing, breathing or movement – for up to 10 seconds. If circulation is active, continue to give 10 breaths/minute, checking for circulation every minute.

- If the casualty starts breathing spontaneously but remains unconscious, place them in the recovery position.

- If you are not successful in achieving effective breaths or if signs of circulation are absent, start chest compressions (SEE *page 340*).

For babies and children aged 1–7

- For children aged 1–7, use the same method as for an adult but at 20 breaths/minute rather than 10.

- For a baby below 1 year, cover both their nose and mouth with your lips or breathe into their nose. Give 20 breaths/minute.

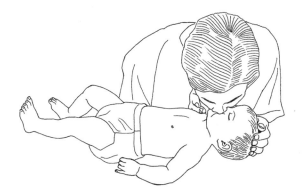

Chest Compressions

CALL AN AMBULANCE.

CPR is designed to resuscitate an unconscious casualty who has stopped breathing and has no circulation. Circulation is necessary because vital organs such as the brain and heart require a constant supply of oxygen to avoid irreversible injury. Some circulation can be achieved artificially by means of chest compressions, which enable the heart to pump the blood around the body. Chest compressions are always used together with rescue breathing (SEE *pages 337–9*) so that the blood receives a supply of oxygen.

- Kneeling beside the casualty, place the middle and index fingers of one of your hands on the notch at the base of the breastbone.

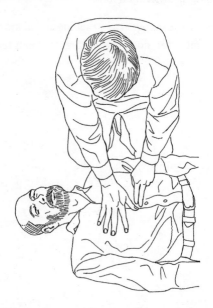

- Place the heel of your other hand on the breastbone next to your fingers – this is where to apply the chest compressions.

- Remove your first hand and rest
  its heel on top of the second
  hand. Lock the fingers of the
  upper hand firmly between
  the fingers of the lower
  hand.

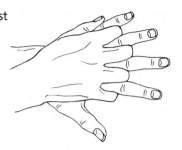

- Lean over the casualty with straight arms and press downwards on
  their breastbone, depressing the chest about 4–5 cm (1½–2 inches).
  Release the pressure, still keeping your hands in place. Perform
  fifteen of these compressions at a rate of 100/minute, followed by
  two rescue breaths. Continue sequences of fifteen compressions
  followed by two rescue breaths until help arrives or the casualty
  moves or takes a breath on their own.

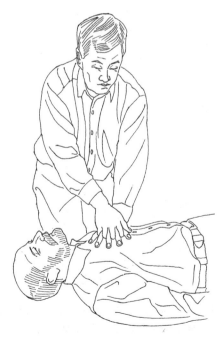

Chest compressions for children aged 1–7 years

● Place the heel of one of your hands on their lower breastbone and perform five chest compressions to one rescue breath.

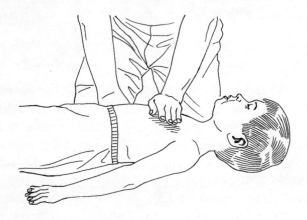

Chest compressions for babies

● For a baby under one year, place two fingers just below the centre point between the nipples and perform five chest compressions to one rescue breath.

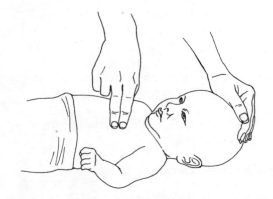

▪ Cuts, Grazes, Splinters

Small cuts, grazes and splinters are minor injuries, but first aid measures are needed to prevent infection, especially tetanus, due to bacteria commonly found in the environment, which can prove fatal.

Small nicks and cuts in the skin may bleed quickly for a few minutes before stopping spontaneously. Grazes are often more painful and more likely to contain dirt, dust and other debris. Splinters can prick intensely yet remain invisible to the naked eye and/or be impossible to squeeze to the skin's surface. Others can remain undetected until the surrounding area becomes inflamed and sore.

Most people are immunized against tetanus during childhood, but may require boosters later on. Seek medical advice if you are not certain of the date of your last immunization or if more than 10 years have elapsed.

WHAT YOU CAN DO

- Wash your hands thoroughly or wear disposable gloves.

- For a small cut or graze, press a clean gauze pad firmly onto the wound and elevate the injured part to above heart level if possible to reduce blood flow.

- Rinse the wound in cold running water. Use a clean gauze pad to coax out any debris and clean the surrounding skin.

- Pat the area dry and apply a little Hypercal (hypericum + calendula) cream.

- Cover with adhesive dressing.

- For a splinter, wash the surrounding area with warm soapy water and pat dry with clean pad.

- Sterilize small tweezers in a flame. Allow to cool.

- Squeeze the surrounding skin to make the splinter stick out and gently extract it with the tweezers in line with the angle of entry.

- Bathe the wound with water containing 2–3 drops of tea tree oil.

- Pat dry. Cover with an adhesive dressing.

SEE YOUR DOCTOR IF...

- You are not currently covered for tetanus immunization.
- The area becomes inflamed, swells or produces pus.
- You become feverish and unwell.
- The whole splinter and/or other debris cannot be removed.

▪ Electric Shock and Burns

CALL AN AMBULANCE.

Major electrical shocks can kill (electrocution); more minor ones can stop a person's breathing, interfere with the heart's rhythm and cause burns. The domestic supply can deliver a fatal shock and 110 volts are particularly likely to trigger cardiac arrhythmia. However, first aid measures can bring very effective help to victims.

WHAT YOU CAN DO

- If the victim is still in contact with the electricity source, take very great care to protect yourself while aiding them. Switch off the supply as close to the main power line as possible, even if fuses and circuit breakers have blown. If this is not possible, push the casualty away from the electricity source using some form of non-conducting or insulated object such as a wooden broom handle, a wooden bench or chair, or a walking stick with no metallic parts. Metal and water are the best electricity conductors, so avoid anything wet or damp – your hands, the floor, even a damp tea towel or oven gloves. If you can, put on rubber gloves and/or stand on a rubber mat or rubber-backed carpet while making your rescue attempt.

- High-voltage electricity carried by rail lines or cables, power lines and commercial generators usually causes instant death. Don't even go near a victim until you are told that it is safe to do so – electricity can arc several metres through the air.

- Once you have switched off the power supply and/or separated the casualty from the faulty appliance, check their breathing and pulse, place them in the *recovery position* and monitor their level of consciousness, breathing and pulse. Loosen their clothing to facilitate *CPR* if necessary.

- Depending upon the condition of the casualty and whether you are alone or someone else is there to aid you, look for burn injuries located at the point at which the current entered and exited the body. These are nearly always more serious than they appear, since much of the damage occurs below the skin. Use the same methods to cool these burns as for other burns (SEE *Burns and Scalds*) and call an ambulance.

■ Eye Injury

WHAT YOU CAN DO

- Examine the eye carefully – if merely bruised, i.e. 'black', make a *cold compress*, adding a drop or two of Arnica tincture to the water, and apply it to the bruise for 15 minutes. If both eyes are black, a head injury may be responsible (SEE *Unconsciousness*).

- A speck of debris floating on the white of the eye can be removed with gently running water, then the eye bathed with hypericum and calendula solution. Larger objects can sometimes be dabbed off the eyeball, lifting the upper lid if necessary, using a piece of sterile gauze or clean handkerchief dipped in the same solution.

- For bad cuts or bruises and penetrating objects such as glass or splinters, call for medical help and lie the casualty down. Place a pad over both eyes, ask them to hold it in place and rest their head on your lap. Hold their head gently while waiting for help.

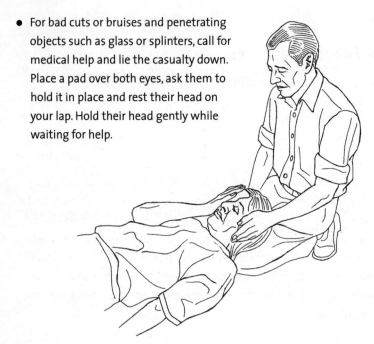

For chemicals in the eye

- Chemicals must be removed urgently. Wear protective gloves if available and hold the casualty's head under a cold running tap for at least 10 minutes so that the eye is thoroughly rinsed. Ensure that contaminated water runs away freely, without touching the other eye or the rest of the face. If both eyes are affected, treat each in turn.

- Once the pain has eased, place two drops of Bach Rescue Remedy on the casualty's tongue. Place a sterile dressing or clean handkerchief lightly over the eye and bandage loosely in place.

- Send/take the casualty to hospital. Make a note of the chemical involved if at all possible.

▪ Febrile Seizures

CALL AN AMBULANCE IF THE CHILD LOSES CONSCIOUSNESS, EVEN BRIEFLY.

Febrile convulsions are relatively common in children aged 1–4 years. They are caused by a high temperature, for example due to a throat infection. The eyes of the hot, flushed, sweaty child may roll backwards in their head and they may arch their back and clench their fists. *Unconsciousness* may follow and the child's body may twitch and shake. These seizures can last from a few seconds to a minute or so and the chief need is to cool the child down while preventing injury. Medical advice should be sought (even if consciousness is not lost) to eliminate more serious causes for the convulsion.

WHAT YOU CAN DO

- Place cushions, pillows, blankets, etc. around the child to prevent physical harm. Avoid restraining or moving the child while in convulsion and never put anything into their mouth.

- To lower the child's temperature, undress them down to their pants and open a window or door to let in some cool air.

- When the convulsion stops, lie the child on their side and cover them with a sheet or light blanket. When they are fully conscious, give them the recommended dose of paracetamol (if they are your own). Seek medical advice.

- For loss of consciousness, place the child in the *recovery position*, call an ambulance and regularly record the pulse, respiration and level of response.

▪ Fractures and Dislocations

GET MEDICAL ATTENTION AT ONCE.

A fracture is a crack or break in a bone, usually resulting from a fall, blow or wrench. The majority of fractures are 'closed', i.e. the skin remains unbroken, but in an 'open' fracture, the fragmented bone protrudes through the skin. Fractures of major bones such as the femur, or thigh bone, can result in *shock* and serious internal bleeding. When a joint is dislocated, its bony components are pulled out of normal alignment. Both types of injury cause local pain, swelling, *bruising* and deformity, and will severely restrict movement.

WHAT YOU CAN DO

● Place 1–2 drops of Bach Rescue Remedy on the casualty's tongue.

For a broken arm

● If the casualty can bend their arm, ask them to support it. If the bone is protruding, wash your hands or wear gloves and lightly cover the area with a clean dressing. If there is bleeding, apply pressure to stem the flow, avoiding the bone end.

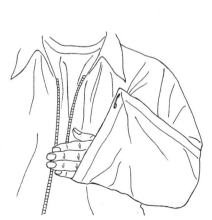

● Make a sling with a triangular bandage or the edge of the casualty's jacket pinned up over the arm to the top of the garment. Don't let them drink, eat or smoke in case they need to have a general anaesthetic later.

● If the arm cannot be bent, lie the casualty down and support the injured elbow with cushions, pillows or other padding.

● Call an ambulance.

For a broken leg

- Support the limb by placing rolled blankets,
  garments or other padding around it.
  Do not allow the casualty to smoke,
  drink or eat in case they need to
  have a general anaesthetic later.

- If the bone is protruding, wash your hands or wear gloves. Lightly
  cover the area with a clean dressing. If there is bleeding, apply
  pressure to stem the flow, avoiding the bone end.

- Call an ambulance.

▪ Insect Bites and Stings

Most bites and stings cause temporary discomfort, but some
people are highly sensitive to them – especially wasp and bee
stings – and develop *anaphylactic shock*, which can prove life-
threatening unless immediately treated.

Bee, wasp and hornet stings can be very painful, however,
and the site of the sting can very quickly become inflamed, hot and
swollen. Many victims suffer more from the fear of the insect

and having been stung than from the inflicted wound, so it is important to calm the casualty to prevent a panic attack. Mosquito bites may not be felt at the time they occur, but can very soon produce intense itching followed by pain in the nearby muscle and skin area.

Ticks, small blood-sucking creatures common in cattle- and sheep-farming country, produce a small round swollen lump on the skin's surface and can cause tick fever, so must be removed as soon as they are spotted.

Fleas have more nuisance than injury value. They cause intense skin irritation, particularly in hot dark warm body areas such as below and between the breasts, around the waist and in the small of the back. They are passed on by cats, dogs and other domestic animals, and stringent measures involving treatment of carpets, bedding, mattresses and soft furnishing (in addition to the pets) are often necessary in order to get rid of a plague of them.

WHAT YOU CAN DO

- Treat an insect sting as soon as possible after it has occurred:

  o If you are stung on your hand, fingers or wrist, remove watches and jewellery in case the area becomes swollen.

  o If the sting is on an arm or leg, raise the limb on a cushion, pillow, etc. to reduce swelling.

  o If you cannot see the sting, wash the area with soap and water and make an ice pack of a cloth soaked in cold water, or crushed ice cubes or frozen vegetables wrapped in a towel. Apply this to the site for at least 10 minutes.

  o If you can see the sting, scrape it out with a firm-edged object such as your fingernail, a coin or an emery board. Avoid using tweezers, as they can squirt more toxin into the sting site.

- To remove a tick, however, you should use tweezers. Grasp the tick's body and manoeuvre it out gently in order to avoid leaving any of its head parts behind. Place it in a bottle, label it and take it to your doctor for identification and any further advice.

- Watch for symptoms of *anaphylactic shock* – call an ambulance if necessary.

- Also call an ambulance if you suspect a sting to the eye, throat or mouth. Apply ice cubes to the site or suck them and sip icy water to allay the symptoms.

- Apply insect bite cream or spray to sore or itchy bites. Avoid scratching because this increases the risk of infection.

- Take an antihistamine tablet (or a brief course) to minimize the swelling and irritation. If assisting a casualty, advise them to seek medical attention and request their own prescription.

▪ Knocked-out Tooth

Children are the most common victims of knocked-out tooth injury. Fights, rough and tumble games, falls from trees and bicycles, car accidents and contact sports can all be responsible. Try to ensure that your child wears appropriate protective clothing, for example a mouth guard, when playing contact sports and strap them securely into an age-appropriate car seat or make certain their seatbelt is properly fastened before undertaking car journeys.

A baby tooth does not need to be repositioned in the mouth as it will be replaced naturally by a permanent tooth later, but a knocked-out permanent tooth is a dental emergency. Returning the stray tooth to its socket as quickly as possible is key to preserving it. Every minute a tooth is out of its socket reduces its chance of survival – stray teeth returned within 30 minutes of the accident stand the best chance.

WHAT YOU CAN DO

- Find the missing tooth. Handle it only by its crown (top white part), never by its root. Gently rinse it in saline (salt and water) solution or milk (do not pick at or scrub it) and use tap water only if you have to – the chlorine could damage the live root.

- Prevent the tooth from drying out while you contact a dentist by:

  ○ Inserting it into its socket (providing, in the case of a child, that they are old enough and calm enough to hold it in place).

  ○ Storing it in milk (not water) or placing it between your teeth and lower gum.

■ The Recovery Position

This position is for an unconscious but still breathing casualty from the age of one year upwards. It prevents them from choking on vomit or their tongue and keeps them in a stable position while you wait for help to arrive.

The following procedure is for a casualty lying on their back. If they are on their front or side, adapt it accordingly.

- Remove any spectacles or objects such as bunches of keys or mobile phones which may hinder you as you move the casualty.

- Take the arm of the casualty that is lying nearer to you and place it at right angles to their body, palm upwards, with the elbow bent.

- Take the casualty's further hand, bring it across their chest and hold it against their cheek.

- Take hold of the thigh further away from you and pull it towards you so that the casualty rolls over towards you and comes to rest lying on their side.

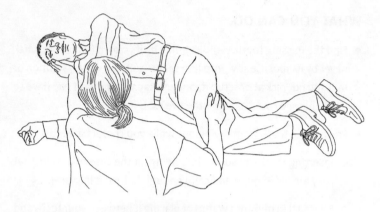

- Take their upper leg and move it so that the hip and knee are at right angles and the knee is supporting the body.

- Move the head back slightly to keep the airway free. If necessary, move the hand that is below the cheek to support the head.

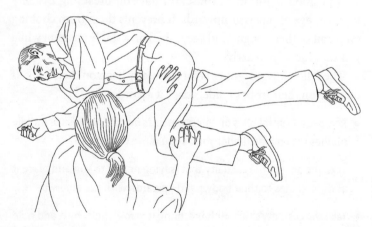

For babies

- When dealing with an
  unconscious but
  breathing baby under
  one year, ensure that the
  airway is open then cradle
  the baby in your arms with
  their head downwards.
  This position keeps
  their airway open.

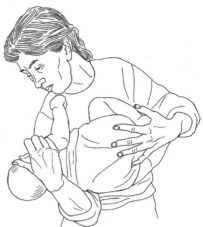

- When dealing with an unconscious but breathing baby over one
  year, ensure that the airway is open then follow the steps described
  above for an adult.

■ Seizures

CALL AN AMBULANCE if you are unclear whether this is the
casualty's first seizure, if *unconsciousness* lasts for more than 10
minutes or if the casualty convulses for more than 5 minutes or
suffers repeated seizures.

During a sudden seizure, convulsion or fit, a person may cry
out, drop to the ground, urinate, go rigid, arch their back and
shake convulsively. Loss of consciousness, either partial or total,
will result.

Epilepsy is the most common cause of a seizure, but head
injuries, alcoholic or other drug poisoning and certain brain
disorders can all be responsible. High temperatures are frequently
the cause in children (SEE *Febrile Seizures*). Seizures can be

frightening to watch, but they usually stop after a few minutes and do not cause lasting injury.

WHAT YOU CAN DO

- If forewarned of an attack, stand behind the casualty and try to ease their fall. Remove sharp objects such as cutlery and scalding drinks that may be nearby and place them out of reach. Never place objects in the casualty's mouth or try to prevent their convulsive movements. Give the casualty space by asking others to stand out of the way.

- Note when the seizure started so you can time its length.

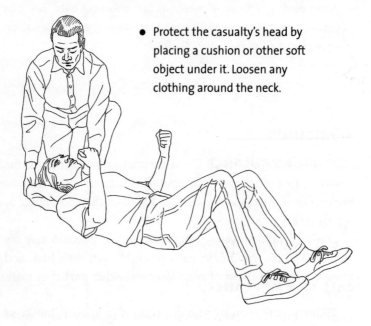

- Protect the casualty's head by placing a cushion or other soft object under it. Loosen any clothing around the neck.

- After the seizure, the casualty may fall asleep. If they are breathing, place them in the *recovery position* and record their levels of response, breathing and pulse until they wake. If they stop breathing, call an ambulance and be ready to start *CPR*.

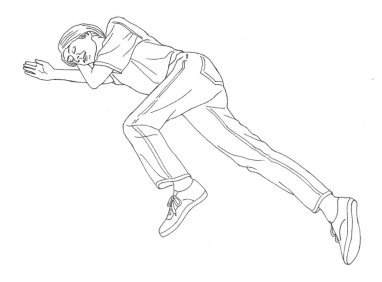

- If it is not necessary to call an ambulance, stay with the casualty until they have completely recovered, then arrange for them to go home and advise them to contact their doctor.

■ Severe Bleeding

CALL AN AMBULANCE.

Common causes of severe bleeding include industrial and work-related accidents, stab wounds and deep cuts. It is vital to stem the blood flow and monitor the casualty's condition to prevent them from developing life-threatening *shock*.

WHAT YOU CAN DO

- While awaiting medical help, wash your hands or wear disposable gloves, then apply pressure to the wound with the palm of your hand or a clean non-fluffy pad to stem the blood flow.
  If an object is embedded in the wound, do not extract it, but press firmly on either side to bring the edges of the wound together.

- Help the casualty to lie down, but keep the injured area elevated above heart level to reduce the bleeding. Press on the wound firmly for 10 minutes.

- Once the bleeding slows, cover the wound with a sterile dressing or clean pad. Bandage it firmly enough to keep the dressing in place but not so tightly as to restrict the circulation. NB Do not apply a tourniquet. Avoid pressing on any embedded object – build up the padding and bandage on either side.

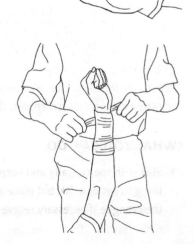

- If bleeding continues, apply a second dressing. If seeping continues, remove both and apply a fresh one. Bandage firmly, applying pressure on the wound.

- To check the circulation, press on a nail or skin beyond the bandage every 10 minutes. Release it when it turns pale. If the colour fails to return, or does so slowly, the bandage is too tight – loosen it slightly.

- If the casualty is fully conscious, place 2–3 drops of Bach's Rescue Remedy on their tongue.

- Record their breathing, pulse and consciousness level regularly. Remain alert for signs of *shock* and if necessary lift their legs above heart level to aid the blood's return to the heart and head. If the casualty loses consciousness, be ready to apply *CPR*.

▪ Shock

CALL AN AMBULANCE AT ONCE.

Shock is a potentially fatal condition in which the blood circulation fails, depriving the brain, heart and other vital organs of oxygen and glucose. *Severe bleeding* is usually responsible, but other causes include loss of body fluids secondary to severe *burns*. The warning signs are a fast pulse, sweating and pale clammy skin. These are succeeded by a weak pulse, shallow, rapid breathing, thirst, restlessness and weakness. The casualty may lose consciousness. Without treatment, their heart will stop.

WHAT YOU CAN DO

- Stay with the casualty and keep them still. Do not give them anything to eat or drink, but place a drop of Bach's Rescue Remedy on their tongue. If necessary, relieve thirst by moistening their lips with a little water.

- Treat any obvious cause for shock such as *severe bleeding* or *burns* (remember that bleeding may be internal, for example following a road accident or *fracture*).

- Loosen the casualty's clothing at the neck, waist and chest. Lie them down on a blanket and, if their legs are uninjured, lift them up onto a stool or cushions to aid the blood's return to the heart and head.

- Cover them with a coat or blanket to keep them warm.

- Regularly record their breathing, pulse and consciousness level. If they lose consciousness, be ready to start *CPR*.

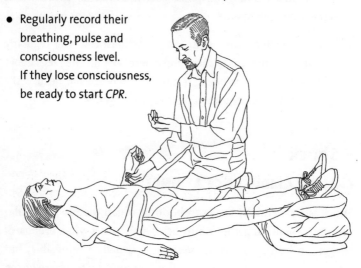

▪ Spinal Injuries

CALL AN AMBULANCE.

Spinal injuries are not uncommon and you should suspect them if the casualty has fallen from a height, fallen awkwardly while doing gymnastics or trampolining, or dived into a shallow pool and hit the bottom. Other familiar scenarios include horse-riding accidents, road traffic accidents involving sudden deceleration or in which the casualty has been flung or tossed in the air, being in a collapsed rugby scrum and receiving a blow to the head or face.

Injury to the spinal cord can occur without the vertebrae being damaged, but spinal *fracture* greatly increases the risks. The most vulnerable spinal areas are those of the neck and lower back, and symptoms suggestive of bony damage include a hollow, twist or irregularity in the spine's normal contours, pain in the neck or back at the site of injury and tender skin overlying the spine. Symptoms indicating spinal cord injury include loss of bladder or bowel function, breathing difficulties, weak or absent limb movements and loss of or altered sensation such as pins and needles and burning. The limbs may feel heavy, stiff or clumsy.

WHAT YOU CAN DO

If the casualty is conscious

- Do not move them unless they are in danger. Reassure them and ask them to keep still.

- Kneel behind the casualty's head. Grasp the sides of their head firmly, with your hands over their ears, while still allowing them to hear you. Steady and support their head in the neutral (i.e. least harmful) head position, in which head, neck and spine are aligned.

- Continue to support their head in the neutral position until the emergency services take over. If available, get help to monitor and record their level of consciousness, pulse and breathing.

- If you suspect a neck injury, ask a helper to place rolled-up blankets, towels or clothing on either side of casualty's head while maintaining it in the neutral position. Continue to support the head and neck throughout until the emergency services arrive.

If the casualty is unconscious

- Kneel behind the casualty and support their head in the neutral position as for a conscious patient.

- If necessary, open the casualty's airway. Place your hands on either side of their face with your fingertips at the angles of the jaws. Gently lift the jaw to open the airway, being careful not to tilt the head.

- Check the casualty is breathing. If so, continue to support their head. If you are alone and need to leave them to call the emergency services, and if they are unable to maintain an open airway, turn them into *the recovery position* before you leave.

- If the casualty is not breathing and there are no signs of circulation, give rescue breaths and chest compressions (SEE *CPR*). Regularly record the level of consciousness, pulse and breathing rate until help arrives.

Log-rolling technique

- This is for use when moving a casualty with a spinal injury. Ideally you should have five helpers, but you can manage with three. Support the casualty's head and neck and ask your helpers to straighten their limbs gently. Then, working in unison, direct your helpers to roll the casualty. Keep their head, trunk and toes in a straight line throughout the manoeuvre.

▪ Sprains and Strains

SEE 'What you Can Do' in *Sprains and Strains*, pages 303–4.

The RICE Procedure

RICE stands for Rest, Ice, Compression and Elevation:

- **Rest** the injured limb or body part (for example, if you have strained a back muscle) in as comfortable a position as possible. Avoid any movement or activity which triggers or aggravates the pain.

- **Ice** will reduce the swelling and relieve the pain. Apply an ice pack to the injury if you keep one in the freezer for emergencies or use a bag of frozen vegetables or some crushed ice cubes wrapped in a cloth. You can also soak a cloth in cold water and lay that over the sprain, adding a few drops of Arnica or Comfrey tincture if available. Leave it in place for 10 minutes.

- **Compression** means applying firm but gentle pressure to the area. First of all place a sterile pad or dressing over the injury, then use an elasticated bandage to keep it in place and apply the pressure. Check that it is not too tight by pressing a nail or skin area beyond the bandage until it turns pale, then releasing it. If the colour does not return quickly, the circulation is being restricted. Loosen the bandage slightly.

- **Elevation** – raising the injured limb will reduce the blood flow to the area and minimize *bruising*. Rest the limb on a pillow or cushioned stool.

- Place a drop or two of Bach's Rescue Remedy onto the casualty's tongue to minimize *shock*.

■ Unconsciousness

CALL AN AMBULANCE.

An unconscious casualty does not react to being shaken or to loud noises and neither moves nor makes any sound. Their eyes may be closed and they may vomit, making lying on their back potentially life-threatening. Common causes include *severe bleeding*, shock, head injuries, *spinal injuries*, poisoning, *choking* and other breathing difficulties.

WHAT YOU CAN DO

- Speak to the casualty loudly and clearly to see whether there is any response. Shake their shoulders very gently in case they have a neck injury (tap a child's shoulder of an infant's foot). If they respond, give first aid to any injuries.

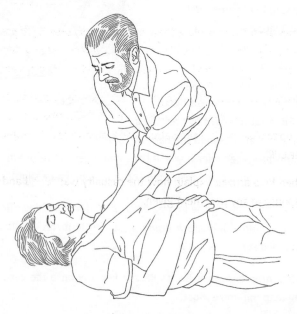

- If there is no response, call for help (if applicable). Place a hand on the casualty's forehead and gently tilt their head backwards to open up their airway. Remove any debris from their mouth and lift their chin. Check their breathing for 10 seconds.

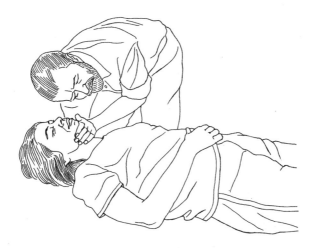

- If they are breathing, place them in *the recovery position*. If possible, treat any obvious injuries like *fractures* or *severe bleeding*. Regularly record their level of response, pulse and breathing until help arrives.

- If they aren't breathing, give two effective rescue breaths (SEE *CPR*) and check for signs of circulation (coughing, movement, breathing) for up to 10 seconds. If circulation is absent, start chest compression (SEE *CPR*).

- When help arrives, explain how the casualty was found and their response to any treatment given.

Glossary of Acupressure Points

For further information on the location of acupressure points, see *Resources and Further Reading.*

Abdominal Sorrow – below the edge of the rib cage half an inch in from the line of the nipple.

Bigger Rushing – on the top of the foot in the valley between the big toe and second toe.

Bigger Stream – in the hollow between the protrusion of the inside ankle bone and the Achilles tendon (which runs from the calf muscle to the back of the heel).
CAUTION: do not stimulate this point after the third month of pregnancy.

Bubbling Springs – at the base of the ball of the foot, between the two toe pads.

Calf's Nose – just below the kneecap in the outer indentation.

Commanding Middle – in the centre of the back of the knee, in the crease of the joint.

Crooked Pond – on the top, outer end of the elbow crease.

Ding Chuan – to each side and slightly above the vertebra that protrudes at the top of the spine when the head is tilted downwards.

Drilling Bamboo – in the indentation outside of the bridge of the nose on the inner edge of the eyebrows.

Ear Gate – half an inch below **Listening Place**.

Elegant Mansion – in the hollow below the collarbone, next to the breastbone.

Eyes Bright – in the hollow in the inner corner of the eye, just above the tear duct.

Facial Beauty – at the bottom of the cheekbone directly below the pupil of the eye.

Four Whites – one finger's width below the lower ridge of the eye socket, in line with the pupil in an indentation of the cheek.

Gates of Consciousness – just below the base of the skull, in the hollow between the two large neck muscles, 2–3 inches apart depending on the size of the head.

Grandfather, Grandson – within the arch of the foot one thumb width from the ball of the foot.

Great Abyss – in the groove at the wrist fold below the base of the thumb.

Heaven Rushing Out – at the base of the throat in the large hollow directly below the Adam's Apple.

Heavenly Pillar – half an inch below the base of the skull, on the rope of muscle half an inch out from either side of the spine.

Heavenly Rejuvenation – on the shoulders, midway between the base of the neck and the outer aspect of (each) shoulder, half an inch below the top of the shoulder.

Inner Gate – in the middle of the inner side of the forearm, two and a half finger widths from the crease of the wrist.

Intermediary – four finger widths above the centre of the inner wrist crease, between the tendons.

Jaw Chariot – between the upper and lower jaw on the (masseter) muscle, which bulges when the back teeth are clenched.

Joining the Valley – in the webbing between the thumb and index finger at the highest spot of the muscle, which becomes prominent when these two digits are brought together.

Jumping Circle – in the centre of the buttock, in the most prominent part of the upper thigh bone.

Listening Place – directly in front of the ear opening in an indentation, which is more noticeable when the mouth is opened.

Lung Associated Point – one finger's width below the upper tip of the shoulder blade, between the spine and the shoulder blade.

Middle of a Person – two-thirds of the way between the centre of the upper lip and the nose.

Outer Arm Bone – on the outer surface of the upper arm, one-third of the way down from the top of the shoulder. (Locate a tough muscular band by rubbing the forefinger over the bone on the outside of the arm.)

Reunion of Hearing – half an inch below **Listening Place**.

Sea of Energy – two finger widths directly below the navel.

Sea of Tranquillity – on the midline of the breastbone, three thumb widths up from the base of that bone.

Sea of Vitality – in the lower back between the second and third lumbar vertebrae, two to four finger widths apart at waist level. CAUTION: do not press on diseased discs, or diseased or fractured bones. If you have a back problem, either avoid this point, or apply light touching for a few minutes.

Severe Mouth – on the outside of the base of the nail of the second toe.

Shoulder Well – on the highest point of the shoulder muscle midway between the outer tip of the shoulder and the spine. CAUTION: pregnant women should press this point lightly.

Third Eye Point – midway between the eyebrows at the junction of the bridge of the nose and the forehead.

Three Mile Point – four finger widths below the kneecap, one finger's width outside the shin bone.

Vital Diaphragm – between the shoulder blade and the spine, at the level of the heart.

Welcoming Perfume – just to the side of the nostril opening.

Wind Screen – in the hollow behind the ear lobe.
CAUTION: press gently as this is a tender and delicate area.

Womb and Vitals – two finger widths outside the widest portion of the sacrum, the flat bone at the base of the spine at the level of the jutting hipbone.

Resources and Further Reading

Useful Websites

- **Acupressure: www.dishant.com/acupressure** provides information on current research into acupressure including the connections between acupressure and neurophysiology.

- **Arthritis Care: www.arthritiscare.org.uk**; tel: 020 7380 6500; fax: 020 7380 6505. This is the largest voluntary organization working with and for people with arthritis.

- **Arthritis Research Campaign: www.arc.org.uk**. Visit this website to find out the latest research into the condition.

- **Back Care: www.backcare.org.uk** provides information about the causes and treatments of back pain. Back Care's Helpline: 0870 950 0275 (national rate).

- **Dementia: www.dementia.com** provides information on memory disorders, Alzheimer's disease and senile dementia. Details of diagnosis, help, medication and news on recent research can be found on this website.

- **Fibromyalgia Association UK: www.fibromyalgia-association uk.org.** The charity offers support and advice for sufferers and their families plus medical information for healthcare professionals.

- **IBS Network: www.ibsnetwork.org.uk.** The network aims to support and educate sufferers of irritable bowel syndrome and their families and carers. For more information call the helpline: 0114 272 3253 (Mon–Fri 6 p.m.–8 p.m. and Sat. 10 a.m.–12 noon).

- **International Menopause Society: www.imsociety.org.** Visit the site to find out more about research into all aspects of ageing in men and women.

- **ME: www.nmec.org.uk** is a useful resource for finding out more about the condition, its treatment and a list of support groups.

- **Menopause Matters: www.menopausematters.co.uk.** Established by clinicians, this site provides information about the symptoms of menopause and treatment options.

- **National Association for Colitis and Crohn's Disease (NACC): www.nacc.org.uk.** For more information call 0845 130 2233 or 0845 130 3344 (NACC-in-Contact support line).

- **Nutrition Matters: www.nutrition-matters.co.uk.** The site has a library with information on specific nutrients and medical conditions as well as up-to-date research.

Information on supplements

- Pumpkin seed oil can be purchased as capsules from most health food stores or it can be mail-ordered from Mortimer and Bennett. For more information, contact Mortimer and Bennett on 020 8995 4145. Alternatively, e-mail **info@mortimerandbennett.com**

- Gengigel is the brand name for hyaluranon, which is available as a gel for application to the gum, or as a liquid for rinsing. Gengigel can be purchased from most dentists, pharmacies and major supermarkets.

Further Reading

Dr Andrew Lockie, *The Family Guide to Homeopathy: The Safe Form of Medicine for the Future*, Hamish Hamilton, London, 1998

Swami Sivananda Radha, *Kundalini Yoga for the West: A Foundation for Character Building, Courage and Awareness*, Timeless Books, Toronto, 1994

Index

Bold entries refer to ailments discussed in Part II.

Order further titles from Robinson

Buy two titles at the offer price and get the cheapest book ½ price
All titles are in the *Daily Telegraph* series

Title	RRP	Offer price	No. of copies	Total
Alzheimer's Disease	£7.99	£6.98		
Chronic Pain	£7.99	£6.98		
Crohn's Disease & Ulcerative Colitis	£9.99	£8.98		
Depression	£9.99	£8.98		
Epilepsy	£9.99	£8.98		
Food Medicine	£9.99	£8.98		
Hip Replacement	£9.99	£8.98		
Learning and Attention Disorders	£7.99	£6.98		
Menopause	£9.99	£8.98		
Migraine	£7.99	£6.98		
Overcoming & Preventing Heart Problems	£9.99	£8.98		
Parkinson's Disease	£9.99	£8.98		
Prostate Disorders	£7.99	£6.98		
Sleep Really Well	£9.99	£8.98		
Stroke	£9.99	£8.98		
A Survival Guide to Later Life	£9.99	£8.98		
P&P & Insurance				£3.00
Grand Total (Please calculate your 50% discount on your second book)				£

Name: _____

Address: _____

_____ Postcode: _____

Daytime Tel. No. / E-mail _____

Three ways to pay:

1. **For express service telephone the TBS order line on 01206 255 800 and quote 'BPHD'. Order lines are open Monday–Friday 8:30a.m.–5:30p.m.**

2. I enclose a cheque made payable to **TBS Ltd** for £ _____

3. Please charge my ☐ Visa ☐ Mastercard ☐ Amex ☐ Switch (switch issue no. ......) £ _____

   Card number: _____

   Expiry date: _____ Signature _____
   (your signature is essential when paying by credit card)

Please return forms (*no stamp required*) to, Constable & Robinson Ltd, FREEPOST NAT6619, 3 The Lanchesters, 162 Fulham Palace Road, London W6 9BR. All books subject to availability.

Enquiries to: readers@constablerobinson.com
www.constablerobinson.com

Constable & Robinson Ltd (directly or via its agents) may mail or phone you about promotions or products. Tick box if you do <u>not</u> want these from us ☐ or our subsidiaries ☐